THE PHYTOGENIC HORMONE SOLUTION

W9-AGZ-186

THE PHYTOGENIC HORMONE
SOLUTION

Restoring Your Delicate Balance with Compounded Natural Hormones

Saundra McKenna, C.N.M.

VILLARD

NEW YORK

Readers are advised to consult a health care provider knowledgeable in alternative/complementary/preventive medicine regarding the prescription dosages, vitamins, minerals, and food supplements that would be beneficial for their particular health needs. Also, if you are using any medications, or if you have any serious health conditions, you must consult with your physician and pharmacist to determine if any vitamin, mineral, phytochemical, herb, juice, or food may be contraindicated. Names have been changed to protect the privacy of the patients whose stories are shared in this book.

Copyright © 2002 by Saundra Koke McKenna, C.N.M.

All rights reserved under International and Pan-American Copyright Conventions. Published in the United States by Villard Books, a division of Random House, Inc., New York, and simultaneously in Canada by Random House of Canada Limited, Toronto.

VILLARD and "V" CIRCLED Design are registered trademarks of Random House, Inc.

Library of Congress Cataloging-in-Publication Data

McKenna, Saundra.
The phytogenic hormone solution : restoring your delicate balance with compounded natural hormones / Saundra McKenna.
p.   cm.
Includes bibliographical references and index.
ISBN 0-8129-9196-6 (trade pbk.)
1. Phytoestrogens.   2. Menopause—Hormone therapy.   3. Plant hormones.
4. Endocrine gynecology.   I. Title.
RG186 .M36   2002
618.1—dc21   2002033097

Villard Books website address: www.villard.com

Printed in the United States of America

24689753

First Edition

Book design by Casey Hampton

This book is dedicated to all the courageous women who choose to trust their inner truth, open their minds and hearts to embrace transformation, and take actions as their inner wisdom guides them to do so.

ACKNOWLEDGMENTS

I offer my deepest gratitude for the opportunity to write this book for you. The process of birthing it has been a labor of love inspired by my commitment to help restore balance in the feminine paradigm. From the depths of my heart, I extend my appreciation to:

Kit Keith, M.D., my dear friend and former Santa Fe practice partner, who provided me with a cottage for my writing retreat;

Khiyani Hill, another dear friend, who truly sees me for who I am, for her encouragement throughout the process of this writing;

My mother, Marjorie, who trusted me enough many years ago to discontinue taking synthetic hormones and continues to take compounded phytogenic hormones;

My friends, who each offered their unique support during the time of this writing, especially Anne, Barbara, Elaine, Ingrid, Jason, Joseph, Leela, Robin, Susan, and Baba;

The pharmacists at Women's International Pharmacy, who understand the ongoing process of fine-tuning hormonal prescriptions, for their patience and compassion with this process;

All the women with whom I have worked, who shared their experiences and experimented to reestablish their most delicate balance, sometimes in the face of desperate despair and many challenges;

Mary Bahr, my editor, whose astute and valuable skills and insights enhanced the clarity with which I wrote this;

Carol Mann, my agent, without whom this could not have been published;

Byron Katie, through whom I gained a greater understanding of "We begin now";

The Diamondback Rattlesnakes, whose intimate encounter propelled me into an unexpected journey, deepening my awareness of myself, lifting the mind's veils, and helping to catalyze my shift into truly being here now;

The guides and angels who patiently offer their love, forgiveness, protection, and timely interventions.

CONTENTS

INTRODUCTION

Hormones are a hot topic among women today as they search for ways to achieve the delicate balance of body, mind, emotions, and spirit that they need to lead complete and rewarding lives. Hormonal imbalances, which can occur at any age and include the menopausal process, are notorious for interfering with the quality of a woman's life. Because of these imbalances, many women find themselves unable to function normally, to perform their daily tasks with their normal levels of focused clarity. A woman may wonder if she is about to have a coronary as her heart suddenly and wildly races with dramatic palpitations, for no apparent reason. These usually well-coping women find themselves unexpectedly in a puddle of tears one minute or snapping angrily over something insignificant the next. Distracted by these physical and emotional symptoms, some women may begin to feel as if they're losing their minds. And if the woman has a partner, their level of intimacy may not only be interrupted, it may become damaged beyond repair.

As a woman's health practitioner, I have been working with women's hormonal issues since 1986. Most of the women I have treated felt desperate when they came to see me.

They heard about the benefits of hormone replacement therapy (HRT)—that estrogen slows the aging process, prevents Alzheimer's disease, acts as a mood elevator, and protects the heart and bones. Many of them have tried taking synthetic hormones, but they did not feel comfortable with the plethora of side effects and the increased risk of cancer.

Then a major breakthrough in treating hormonally rooted problems occurred when prescribing compounded phytogenic natural hormones became an option. *Phytogenic* hormones, which are compounded in a laboratory from a plant base, are identical to those hormones naturally occurring in a woman's body, and they do not increase the risk for cancer. The compounding process enables precise dosages and potency. Compounded phytogenic natural hormones, administered in NHRT (natural hormone replacement therapy), effectively treat the negative symptoms that arise from this imbalance—promoting optimal immune health, thus helping to prevent Alzheimer's disease and reverse osteoporosis. While *phytohormones* occur naturally in plants and have hormonelike effects in their original state, the precision of strength and effectiveness is unclear.

Women at any age can develop hormonal imbalances. A woman who has just had a baby or a teenager who is beginning to establish her own hormonal rhythm may find herself at the mercy of her hormones. Young women, shocked at the prospect, can find themselves prematurely in the perimenopausal process. Many factors influence that delicate, everchanging balance—stress, illness, travel, and genetics. When we nurture and stabilize our hormones, we not only enhance our ability to function better, but we also free ourselves to focus on our priorities and live life. Band-Aid treatments that simply placate disturbing symptoms do not remedy underlying causes.

I have been prescribing compounded phytogenic hormones since the inception of individualized compounds. And for many years, women have been asking me to write a book on the use of this safe and effective hormone option. These women had had trouble finding adequate information about alternatives to synthetic hormone therapies for such conditions as PMS, acne, endometriosis, uterine fibroids, ovarian cysts, irregular cycles, miscarriages, and the standard HRT (hormone replacement therapy) prescriptions. These women recognized their need for help but were unhappy with what traditional medicine offered them.

No single formula or prescription can elicit the expected change for everyone. There is no generic approach to hormonal balance. There are many variables to consider in finding what constitutes balance for each woman. Because compounded phytogenic hormones do not shut down a woman's own hormonal production—rather, they augment hormones and supplements where there is an insufficiency—the prescriptions need to change over time. Estrogen and progesterone alone are not enough for the women who also need DHEA and testosterone. Nor does every woman need added estrogen. No matter how different we each seem to be, we all want to feel good about our lives. We want to feel beautiful, to love, and be happy. And believe me, a woman with her hormones running amok feels pretty insane. She does not feel good about herself, and thus finds her love of herself and others challenged.

Most symptoms caused by hormonal imbalances can be resolved, but it is important to first understand the nature of a symptom's fundamental cause in order to correct it. With a little patience, clear communication, and recognition of the imbalances, you can restore your body, mind, and spirit's symmetry. You can feel and look like yourself again, perhaps even better.

The Phytogenic Hormone Solution presents stories from among the hundreds of courageous women in my practice who have chosen to experiment with the compounded hormones extracted from plants. I have changed the names of these women to protect their privacy. By sharing their stories, their individualized formulas, and how and why adjustments in their dosages were needed, it is my intention to inspire hope for the many women undergoing any of these hormonal imbalances. These stories illustrate their success in realizing hormonal balance, without increasing the risk for breast, uterine, or ovarian cancer.

Threaded throughout the chapters are examples of the various symptoms of hormonal imbalances. As you relate your own unique experiences to these examples, some extreme, some subtle, you can develop a clearer understanding of your own process. You will find checklists, Rx Summaries, and tools to help you evaluate your relationship to specific hormonal deficiencies. It is my intention to demystify the hormonal quandaries in language every woman can understand.

A NOTE TO THE READER

I realize that many women will turn to the end of each chapter and section for the Rx Summary relating to their specific condition. For a fuller explanation of specific homeopathic, herbal, vitamin and mineral, and aromatherapy remedies, please refer to the Glossary of Remedies in Part Four. A detailed description of a whole-foods diet and an explanation of its benefits are given in Chapter 3.

PART ONE

HORMONES REVEALED

HORMONE THERAPY MYTHOLOGY UNVEILED

WHAT ARE PHYTOGENIC HORMONES?

Let's get the technical data covered and out of the way so we can move on to the issues that concern you the most, your hormonal balance—how to recognize an imbalance, what hormones are responsible, and how to restore your own delicate, ever-changing balance.

The term *phytogenic* literally means *of plant origin*. Hormones, chemical messengers originating in an organ or gland, disperse into the bloodstream to other parts of the body and stimulate chemical reactions to increase functional activity and secretion of the specific hormones. Hormones interact with one another and are responsible for creating and maintaining balance within each of us. The hormonal system performs the most delicate balancing act of all the systems in our bodies. To maintain our stability, we are dependent upon our hormonal balance, which affects us in many aspects of our being human—physically, mentally, emotionally, and even our spiritual sense of well-being, independent of specific belief systems. (Many women have plunged into an existential crisis resulting from hormonal imbalances.) As you will see in the next two parts of the book, when our hormones are out of balance, we do not function well, nor do we as easily retain optimal health. Imbalanced hormones can alter the normal functioning of other systems, eliciting a multitude of challenging symptoms and potentially evolving into disease.

Phytogenic hormones are created from diosgenin, a large steroid molecule that exists in plants such as the Mexican wild yam and soybeans. This molecule, extracted in a laboratory, can be compounded into each specific hormone—estrone, estradiol, estriol, progesterone, testosterone, and DHEA (dehydroepiandrosterone)—to become hormones that are biochemically identical to the hormones our bodies make.

Because these compounded phytogenic hormones are identical to our own, hence the term *bioidentical,* or *human isomolecular,* they are recognized by our endocrine system and accepted alongside our own hormones. Once our natural hormone levels have declined, these hormones maintain the essential hormonal balance we require to feel vital, to function at our optimal levels, and to support our general health and well-being.

Phytohormones are plants that in their natural form of existence have hormonal effects. Many of the available over-the-counter (OTC) natural products designed to assist with the symptoms of PMS, perimenopause, and menopause do not contain any actual hormones. You will see the word *phytohormone* on the label, and the ingredients list will include specific herbs. Or, for example, Promensil by Reach 4 Life states that it contains "40 milligrams of plant estrogen"—this means that plants having 40 mg of estrogenic qualities have been used in the formula. Plant estrogen or progesterone has not been extracted and then converted into actual human, bioidentical estrogen or progesterone. These are quite different from the *phytogenic hormones* that have been compounded into specific amounts of each hormone, which then become bioidentical to human hormones and thereby bioavailable for your endocrine system to utilize.

NATURAL HORMONES DEMYSTIFIED

The term *natural* is applied to all hormones derived from plant extracts, which are thus phytogenic by nature. They are considered natural not because of their natural source but because they are identical to naturally occurring human hormones and because of the way they interact in the human endocrine system. Many products claim to be natural. Actual phytogenic hormones will specify the hormone by name, as in, for example, USP progesterone, rather than plant progesterone.

Extracted from either wild yam or soy, each of the three estrogens—estrone (E1), estradiol (E2), and estriol (E3)—plus progesterone, DHEA, and testosterone can be combined into a specific compound tailored to what each woman needs to feel her best and sustain her hormonal balance. In a triestrogen formula the ratio is, most commonly, 10 percent each of estrone and estradiol and 80 percent estriol, whereas a biestrogen formula is 20 percent estradiol, 80 percent estriol, and excludes estrone completely. Estrone is the primary circulating estrogen in most postmenopausal women. These ratios can be altered as needed to facilitate a more positive response.

Phytogenic progesterone, most commonly extracted from the Mexican wild yam, can be taken alone or in combination with any of the other hormones that a woman needs to restore balance. There are many types of progesterone in creams and sublingual sources now available over the counter. The disadvantage with many of these nonprescription progesterones is the lack of clarity in the exact amounts contained in each dosage. If it does not state on the label the number of milligrams in each dose, you do not know how much progesterone you are actually taking. If the label does not specify the word *progesterone* in the ingredients, it lacks any actual progesterone.

As a practitioner, in order to better monitor over time the adjustments a woman needs to restore balance, I want to know exactly how much progesterone she is really taking into her system. If she needs progesterone along with estrogen, testosterone, and/or DHEA, it is less expensive to have a compounding pharmacy put this all into one formula than to use a combination of different nonprescription sources. While experimenting to establish your best dosage, you might want to take each hormone separately until you have continued to take the same amount consistently for several months.

THEY TORTURE HORSES, DON'T THEY?

I invite you to explore the unnecessary process of extracting estrogen from a pregnant mare to produce the most widely and routinely prescribed synthetic estrogen, Premarin. Premarin stands for PREgnant MARes' urINe. What's unnatural about urine? is the common defense for this drug. Urine in and of itself is the result of a natural physiologic process common to every known biological creature on this planet. Urine therapy is not a new concept. In Ayurveda, a specific healing modality thousands of years old, one drinks one's own urine as a remedy to cure disease, as well as to rejuvenate and maintain health.

The problem is that the estrogen found in horse urine is not natural to the human endocrine system. Its molecular structure is quite different from the molecular structure of human estrogens and the estrogens compounded from plant extracts. Premarin contains equine estrogens— estrone and equilin sulfate, equilenin, 17 a-dihydroequilin, 17 a-estradiol, 17 a-dihydroequilenin, and numerous other estrogens found in horses— none of which occur naturally in the human female. Premarin, like all substances, is processed by the liver; it has a greater negative impact on the liver than any bioidentical, phytogenic estrogen does.

In addition, the process used to extract this estrogen from the pregnant mare is a cruel, torturous process in which the mare is confined to a standing position devoid of movement in a narrow stall. A horse normally lies down approximately three hours for every twenty-four-hour cycle. Previously, horses were fitted with a catheter in the bladder during the eleven-month pregnancy; now, urine collection devices are used that allow urine to soak the skin of the vulva, sometimes causing severe infections and painful lesions. For more details on the mistreatment of mares resulting from the extraction of equine estrogens from their urine, go to *www.premarin.org*.

RISKS AND SIDE EFFECTS OF SYNTHETIC ESTROGENS

Taken directly from its package insert and its website, *www.premarin.com*, Wyeth-Ayerst, the company marketing Premarin and related HRTs such as Premphase, Prempac, and Prempro, lists the following as risk factors and side effects of its product:

1. Cancer of the uterus and endometrium (the uterine lining)
2. Cancer of the breast
3. Gallbladder disease
4. Abnormal blood clotting
5. Inflammation of the pancreas
6. Endometriosis (growth of endometrial tissue outside the uterus)

7. Cardiovascular disease including myocardial infarction, pulmonary embolism, and venous thromboembolism and thrombophlebitis—highest in the first year of therapy

8. Hypercalcemia (an excessive amount of calcium in the blood)

9. Hepatic adenoma—although benign and rare, these liver tumors can rupture and may cause death through intra-abdominal hemorrhage.

10. Hepatic carcinoma—cancer of the liver

11. Endometrial hyperplasia (excessive proliferation—rapid reproduction—of normal cells in normal tissue arrangement of the uterine lining)

12. Enlargement of uterine fibroids

13. Familiar hyperlipoproteinemia (an increase in the concentration of the three fatty substances in the blood—cholesterol, phospholipid, and triglyceride, combined with plasma proteins)

14. Glucose intolerance

15. Jaundice in women who had jaundice in their pregnancy

16. Congenital defects in the unborn with malignant potential, if taken in pregnancy

17. High blood pressure

As other side effects, Wyeth-Ayerst alerts you to the following:

In your genitourinary system:

1. Breakthrough bleeding, spotting, change in menstrual flow or amenorrhea (absence of menses)

2. Dysmenorrhea (painful periods)

3. PMS

4. Vaginal candidiasis

5. Change in the erosion of the cervix, effecting cervical secretions

6. Cystitis-like (bladder infection) symptoms

7. Genital itching, burning, and irritation

For your breasts, it warns of:

1. Tenderness

2. Enlargement

3. Secretions from the nipples

In your gastrointestinal tract:
1. Nausea and vomiting
2. Abdominal pain, cramps, and bloating
3. Cholestatic jaundice, caused by the arrest of bile excretion
4. Pancreatitis—inflammation of the pancreas
5. Gallbladder disease

For your skin:
1. Chloasma or melasma—discolorations of the skin, which may not go away even after HRT has been discontinued
2. Erythema multiform—a discolored flat patch of skin eruption with dark red elevated areas and erythema nodosum—red and painful nodules on legs, usually associated with rheumatism but can be caused by certain drugs and food poisoning
3. Hemorrhagic eruptions
4. Loss of scalp hair
5. Hirsutism—excessive hair growth, mostly in unwanted places, or appearance of hair in unusual places

Your central nervous system could develop:
1. Headaches and migraines
2. Dizziness
3. Mental depression
4. Chorea—a nervous affliction marked by muscular twitching of limbs or facial muscles

For your eyes:
1. Steepening of corneal curvature
2. Intolerance to contact lenses

And a few miscellaneous ones:
1. Decrease in carbohydrate tolerance
2. Aggravation of porphyria, a metabolic disorder
3. Edema
4. Anaphylactic reactions—a sudden hypersensitive response to a foreign substance with symptoms severe enough to produce shock requiring immediate treatment and which may result in death

5. Weight gain or loss, though I've only seen weight gain
6. Loss of libido

If you have ever been prescribed Premarin, Premphase, Prempac, or Prempro, were these serious risks and side effects explained to you before you were told to take these hormones? Were you informed that you may feel and look like a pregnant mare, as well? If you had been told all of this before you filled that first prescription, would you have gone to the pharmacy or would you have asked for other options?

WHY TAKE HORMONES AT ALL?

Recent studies argue that taking synthetic estrogen actually increases the rate of heart attacks in the first few years before providing any potential added protection. For years, of the various reasons women were given to justify taking HRT, one of the primary incentives was to reduce the risk of heart disease. The good news is that the compounded phytogenic progesterone and estriol help protect cardiac function.

If you are menopausal or postmenopausal and still have a uterus, you may have heard that you must take progestin—a synthetic progesterone—with estrogen to protect against uterine cancer. Yet the latest study says that women who take estrogen without progestin have a lower incidence of breast cancer. If you dig deeper, you'll find that almost all of the published research involves conjugated synthetic estrogens and synthetic progestin. The incongruity of the results of these studies raises suspicions. What is the truth?

Synthetic estrogen shuts down the functioning of a woman's own available hormones, thus increasing her risk for both breast and uterine cancer. The synthetic progestin is not only less effective than natural progesterone, it also causes harmful side effects such as menstrual irregularities, including the cessation of your cycle or an abnormal flow; nausea; depression; weight fluctuations; fluid retention; insomnia; and jaundice. Medroxyprogesterone, one of the synthetic progestins used in conjunction with synthetic estrogens, is cardiotoxic. This means it's not good for your heart. Compounded phytogenic natural progesterone, by contrast, effectively provides cardiac protection; treats PMS, irregular cycles, in-

somnia, depression, fluid retention, infertility, and nausea; and helps prevent breast cancer, fibrocystic breasts, and uterine fibroids, to name a
few benefits.

Over the past few years, estrogen deficiency has been linked to
Alzheimer's disease, a debilitating dementia that occurs in the forty- to
sixty-year-old age group. Alzheimer's takes a relentless and irreversible
course of a few months to years, and leads to the end stage of helplessness. Compounded phytogenic hormones provide hormonal supplementation without the serious and negative side effects of synthetic
hormones.

Osteoporosis is mostly prevented and reversed with adequately absorbed and utilized progesterone and estrogen, along with weight-bearing
exercise, a diet low in animal protein, and supplementation with a
well-absorbed source of sufficient calcium and magnesium. Previously,
women who had a total hysterectomy and oophorectomy—the removal
of the cervix, uterus, fallopian tubes, and both ovaries—were told they
did not need to take progesterone, that is, until the role progesterone
plays in bone marrow production was understood. Here again, phytogenic hormones effectively nourish and protect without risky side effects.

When I began working with compounded phytogenic hormones
many years ago, I gave women with hysterectomies progesterone with
their estrogen. It made sense to me that if our bodies were accustomed
to having both estrogen and progesterone, a woman needed supplementation of both because she no longer produced either on her own. I noticed how much better these women felt, within a reasonably short time,
than did those women who took only conjugated synthetic estrogens or
combinations of synthetic estrogens and progestins. I prescribed compounded estrogens with progesterone out of what seemed to me pure
common sense, even though this was not considered standard practice at
that time. Years later, research emerged suggesting the importance of
progesterone in the prevention and treatment of osteoporosis.

We live in a world that remains highly out of balance, as is evident by
aggressive and often violent behavior worldwide. Planet Earth needs
healing, rebalancing, and where else to begin this process but with ourselves. As we, the feminine aspect of humanity, choose to restore balance
in ourselves in every way available, including our hormonal balance, we

create opportunities to return the Earth's energy and the masculine aspect to the heart. If we are ever to establish peace in our world, we must begin at home, within ourselves. This requires us to choose to confront our fears with love, compassion, and forgiveness, embracing the feminine paradigm of restoring balance.

HORMONE TREATMENT OPTIONS

The charts on the following pages, modeled after the one the Women's International Pharmacy included in their prescriber handout, will clarify the different hormone options available. They show how to take each one, if they are bioidentical to your own hormones, if you require a prescription (Rx) from your practitioner, or if the hormone or formula is available over the counter (OTC). I recommend that you choose a hormonal approach that is bioidentical, but I have listed the other options frequently prescribed so you can know what they are.

In addition to the combination formulas of compounded phytogenic natural hormones noted in the chart, other combinations are created based upon your need. The most effective methods of testing your hormone levels are discussed in the following chapter. For example, your estrogen levels are fine but you are deficient in progesterone and DHEA. Or your twenty-four-hour urine or salivary hormone analysis reveals that you are not only deficient in progesterone but you also need estrogen and your testosterone bottomed out altogether. You want to take only one dose at a time. No problem. The compounding pharmacy, based on the prescription your practitioner gives them, puts each required hormone, in the exact specified amounts of milligrams, into each capsule, gram of cream, or drop of your sublingual dosage.

ORAL PROGESTERONE AND PROGESTINS

PRODUCT NAME/DESCRIPTION (SUPPLIER/MANUFACTURER)	DOSAGES AVAILABLE	BIO-IDENTICAL	AVERAGE DAILY DOSING	RX OR OTC
Prometrium/natural progesterone in peanut oil (Solvay)	100 mg per capsule	Yes	200–300 mg	Rx
Progesterone/natural progesterone in oil, capsules (compounding pharmacy)	25, 35, 50, 75, 100 mg per capsule	Yes	100 mg every 12 hours	Rx
Natural micronized progesterone in vegetable oil (compounding pharmacy)	3.33 mg per drop	Yes	50–100 mg twice daily in sublingual drops	Rx
PhytoProlief/natural progesterone plus herbs (Arbonne International)	20 mg per capsule	Yes	20–100 mg twice daily	OTC
Progesterone Spray/natural progesterone (Biogenesis Laboratories)	960 mg per 10 oz. and 6 mg spray	Yes	2–20 sprays sublingually twice daily	OTC
Cycrin/medroxyprogesterone acetate (ESI Lederle)	2.5, 5, 10 mg	No	2.5 mg daily 5–10 mg daily for 5–10 days	Rx
Aygestin/norethindrone acetate (ESI Lederle)	5 mg	No	2.5–10 mg daily for 5–10 days	Rx
Nor-QD/norethindrone (Watson)	0.35 mg tabs in a 42-day pack	No	0.35 mg per day	Rx
Micronor/norethindrone (Ortho-McNeil)	0.35 mg tabs in a 28-day pack	No	0.35 mg per day	Rx
Megace/megesterol acetate (Bristol-Myers Squibb)	20 and 40 mg	No	40–160 mg per day	Rx
Provera/medroxyprogesterone acetate (MPA) (Pharmacia Upjohn)	2.5, 5, 10 mg	No	Continuous: 2.5 mg daily Cyclic: 5–10 mg for 5–10 days	Rx

TOPICAL PROGESTERONE CREAMS OR GELS

PRODUCT NAME/DESCRIPTION (SUPPLIER/MANUFACTURER)	DOSAGES AVAILABLE	BIO-IDENTICAL	AVERAGE DAILY DOSING	RX OR OTC
Progesterone/natural progesterone P4—cream or gel (compounding pharmacy)	Many, common range is 2–10%	Yes	25–100 mg twice daily	Rx
Pro-Gest/natural progesterone (Transitions for Health, Inc.)	20 mg per ¼ tsp 450 mg per oz progesterone	Yes	¼–½ tsp twice daily	OTC
Progesterone cream (Woman to Woman)	2%	Yes	20–100 mg twice daily	OTC
Natural Progesterone cream (Awakening Woman)	20 mg per dose	Yes	20–100 mg twice daily	OTC
Wild Yam Cream (Meldown International)	6%	Yes	1–2 doses twice daily	OTC
Progesterone Cream (GL Health)	20 mg per dose	Yes	20–100 mg twice daily	OTC
Progesterone Cream (Source Natural)	500 mg per oz	Yes	20–100 mg twice daily	OTC
Progesterone Cream plus Herbs (Tsang Nutrition)	495 mg per oz progesterone	Yes	20–100 mg twice daily	OTC
Progesterone Cream (Young Again Nutrients)	500 mg per oz progesterone	Yes	20–100 mg twice daily	OTC
Renaissance Progesterone Cream (Lipoceutical)	1,500 mg per 2 oz progesterone	Yes	1–10 doses twice daily	OTC
Women's Balance Cream/ natural progesterone plus herbs (Kokoro)	510 mg per oz progesterone	Yes	20–100 mg twice daily	OTC
Progesterone Cream (LifeInBalance.com)	400 mg per oz progesterone	Yes	20–100 mg twice daily	OTC
Renewed Balance (AIM)	750 mg per oz progesterone	Yes	20–100 mg twice daily	OTC

NOTE: Currently, there are many natural progesterone creams on the market. Of the creams available, unfortunately, many do not state the number of milligrams per dose in the product. Without this specific information, I cannot give a recommended dosage and so I am not including them in this list.

In addition to the prescribed progesterone available through compounding pharmacies, the list above gives you an idea of the varied amounts of OTC dosages available on-line for purchase.

ORAL ESTROGENS

PRODUCT NAME/DESCRIPTION (SUPPLIER/MANUFACTURER)	DOSAGES AVAILABLE	BIO-IDENTICAL	AVERAGE DAILY DOSING	RX OR OTC
Biestrogen/20% estradiol (E2) and 80% estriol (E3) in oil, capsules (compounding pharmacy)	Any	Yes	1.25–5 mg twice daily	Rx
Triestrogen/10% estrone (E1), 10% estradiol (E2), 80% estriol (E3) in oil, capsules (compounding pharmacy)	Any	Yes	1.25–5 mg twice daily	Rx
Estradiol (E2) in oil, capsules (compounding pharmacy)	Any	Yes	1 mg twice daily	Rx
Estrace estradiol (E2) (Bristol-Myers Squibb)	0.5, 1, 2 mg	Yes	1 mg daily	Rx
Natural micronized bi- or triestrogen in vegetable oil (compounding pharmacy)	Any	Yes	1.25–5 mg twice daily in sublingual drops	Rx
Premarin/conjugated equine estrogens (CEE) (Wyeth-Ayerst)	0.3, 0.625, 0.9, 1.25, 2.5 mg tablets	No	0.625 mg daily	Rx
Cenestin/conjugated estrogens (Duramed)	0.625 and 0.9 mg	No	0.625–1.25 mg daily	Rx
Ortho-Est/piperazine estrone sulfate, aka estropipate (Women First Healthcare)	0.625 and 1.25 mg tablets	No	0.625 mg daily	Rx
Ogen/estropipate (Pharmacia Upjohn)	0.625, 1.25, 2.5 mg tablets	No	0.625 mg daily	Rx
Menest/esterfied estrogens (Monarch)	0.3, 0.625, 1.25, 2.5 mg tablets	No	0.625 mg daily	Rx
Estratab/esterfied estrogens (Solvay)	0.3, 0.625, 2.5 mg tablets	No	0.625 mg	Rx

NOTE: There are many other bioidentical formulas manufactured by naturopathic pharmaceutical companies. I do not list them because their products can only be ordered and prescribed for you by your licensed practitioner.

COMBINATION ORAL ESTROGEN WITH PROGESTERONE/PROGESTIN

PRODUCT NAME/DESCRIPTION (SUPPLIER/MANUFACTURER)	DOSAGES AVAILABLE	BIO-IDENTICAL	AVERAGE DAILY DOSING	RX OR OTC
Biestrogen—20% estradiol (E2), 80% estriol (E3)—and progesterone in oil, capsules (compounding pharmacy)	Any (combinations vary based on individual Rx)	Yes	Biestrogen: 1.25–5 mg Progesterone: 35–100 mg twice daily	Rx
Triestrogen—10% estrone (E1), 10% estradiol (E2), 80% estriol (E3)—and progesterone in oil, capsules (compounding pharmacy)	Any (combinations vary based on individual Rx)	Yes	Triestrogen: 1.25–5 mg Progesterone: 35–100 mg twice daily	Rx
Natural micronized bi- or triestrogen and progesterone in vegetable oil (compounding pharmacy)	Any (combinations vary based on individual Rx)	Yes	Bi- or triestrogen: 1.25–5 mg Progesterone: 35–50 mg twice daily in sublingual drops	Rx
Prempro/conjugated equine estrogens (CEE) and medroxyprogesterone acetate (MPA) (Wyeth-Ayerst)	0.625 mg E and 2.5 mg MPA or 0.625 mg E and 5 mg MPA	No	1 tablet daily	Rx
Premphase/conjugated equine estrogens (CEE) and MPA (Wyeth-Ayerst)	Biphasic: 0.625 mg E #14 and 0.625 mg E with 5 mg MPA #14	No	1 tablet daily (28-day pack)	Rx

NOTE: DHEA and/or testosterone can be added to prescription compounded combination.

ESTROGEN AND ESTROGEN/PROGESTIN PATCHES

PRODUCT NAME/DESCRIPTION (SUPPLIER/MANUFACTURER)	DOSAGES AVAILABLE	BIO-IDENTICAL	AVERAGE DAILY DOSING	RX OR OTC
Estraderm/estradiol (E2) (Novartis)	0.05 and 0.1 mg per day	Yes	Patch changed twice weekly	Rx
Vivelle/estradiol (E2) (Novartis)	0.0375, 0.05, 0.075, 0.1 mg per day	Yes	Patch changed twice weekly	Rx
Climara/estradiol (E2) (Berlex Laboratories)	0.05, 0.075, 0.1 mg per day	Yes	Patch changed once weekly	Rx
Alora/estradiol (E2) (Proctor & Gamble)	0.05, 0.075, 0.1 mg per day	Yes	Patch changed twice weekly	Rx
Combi Patch/estradiol (E2) and norethindrone (Rhone-Poulenc)	0.05 mg and 0.14 mg 0.05 mg and 0.25 mg per day	Estrogen Yes; Progestin No	Patch changed twice weekly	Rx

ESTROGEN/PROGESTERONE AND ESTROGEN CREAMS/GELS

PRODUCT NAME/DESCRIPTION (SUPPLIER/MANUFACTURER)	DOSAGES AVAILABLE	BIO-IDENTICAL	AVERAGE DAILY DOSING	RX OR OTC
Biestrogen—20% estradiol (E2), 80% estriol (E3)—and progesterone cream or gel (compounding pharmacy)	Any (combinations vary based on individual Rx)	Yes	Biestrogen: 1.25–5 mg Progesterone: 25–100 mg twice daily	Rx
Triestrogen—10% estrone (E1), 10% estradiol (E2), 80% estriol (E3)—and progesterone cream or gel (compounding pharmacy)	Any (combinations vary based on individual Rx)	Yes	Triestrogen: 1.25–5 mg Progesterone: 25–100 mg twice daily	Rx
Estro Pro Cream/triestrogen and progesterone (Longevity Resource International)	Triestrogen and 550 mg per ounce progesterone	Yes	$1/4$–$1/2$ tsp twice daily	OTC
Estradiol (E2) cream or gel (compounding pharmacy)	Any	Yes	0.5–1 mg twice daily	Rx
Estradiol (E3) cream or gel (compounding pharmacy)	Any	Yes	1–3 mg twice daily	Rx
Bi- or triestrogen (E2E3 or E1E2E3) cream or gel (compounding pharmacy)	Any	Yes	1.25–2.5 mg twice daily	Rx

VAGINAL ESTROGENS

PRODUCT NAME/DESCRIPTION (SUPPLIER/MANUFACTURER)	DOSAGES AVAILABLE	BIO-IDENTICAL	AVERAGE DAILY DOSING	RX OR OTC
Estriol cream or nonalcohol gel (compounding pharmacy)	0.5 to 2 mg per gm	Yes	Apply vaginally daily for 2 weeks then every 2–3 days as needed	Rx
Estring vaginal silicone ring/estradiol (Pharmacia Upjohn)	2 mg in silicone polymer ring	Yes	Releases estradiol at a rate of 7.5µg per 24 hours up to 90 days	Rx
Premarin cream/conjugated equine estrogens (Wyeth-Ayerst)	0.625 mg per gm	No	0.5–2 gm daily for 3 weeks, off one week	Rx
Ogen vaginal cream/ estropipate (Pharmacia Upjohn)	1.5 mg per gm	No	2–4 gm daily for 3 weeks, off one week	Rx
Ortho Dienestrol cream/ dienestrol (Ortho)	0.1 mg per gm	No	1–2 applications daily for 1–2 weeks; 1/2–1 application for 1–2 weeks, then 1 application 1–3 times weekly	Rx

TESTOSTERONE ORAL/CREAM/GEL PREPARATIONS

PRODUCT NAME/DESCRIPTION (SUPPLIER/MANUFACTURER)	DOSAGES AVAILABLE	BIO-IDENTICAL	AVERAGE DAILY DOSING	RX OR OTC
Testosterone USP/micronized in oil, capsules (compounding pharmacy)	Any	Yes	2–10 mg daily	Rx
Testosterone USP/micronized in oil (compounding pharmacy)	Any	Yes	2–10 mg daily in sublingual drops	Rx
Estratest, Estratest HS/esterfied estrogens with methyl-testosterone (Solvay)	1.25 mg E and 2.5 mg MT or 0.625 mg E and 1.25 mg MT (HS)	No	1 daily	Rx
Menogen, Menogen HS/esterfied estrogens with methyltestosterone (Breckenridge)	1.25 mg E and 2.5 mg MT or 0.625 mg E and 1.25 mg MT (HS)	No	1 daily	Rx
Methyltestosterone MT (compounding pharmacy)	Any	No	0.25–0.75 mg daily	Rx
Testosterone oral, sublingual, cream or gel (can be added to combination Rx) (compounding pharmacy)	Any	Yes	2.5–20 mg daily	Rx

ILLUMINATING HORMONES

HOW DO I TEST MY HORMONES?

Should you test from your salivary perspective, through your urine, or through your blood? If you choose to evaluate your hormones through blood tests because your insurance pays for it, when do you have your blood drawn? What hormones should you measure? Do you want to evaluate just the follicle stimulating hormone (FSH) and the lutenizing hormone (LH)? If you want to discern hormonal function, measuring the FSH and/or the LH is inadequate. You really need to see the quantified value of each specific hormone: estrone, estradiol, estriol, progesterone, testosterone, DHEA, and perhaps thyroid, adrenals, and corticosteroid levels as well.

BLOOD TESTING

Blood tests only measure the hormone levels at the time your blood is drawn, and personally, in general, I find they yield less information at a greater cost. Traditionally, the most common blood test ordered to evaluate a woman's hormones has been the FSH and LH to assess ovarian function. If these results measure within the normal range, the woman is told her hormones are fine and normal, even though she's exhibiting symptoms of significant hormonal imbalances. Both the follicle stimulating hormone (FSH) and the lutenizing hormone (LH) are required to stimulate follicle development and estradiol synthesis. Circulating levels of FSH and LH are measurable throughout the cycle and are useful along with measuring all the hormones, especially when working with fertility issues.

Many women have normal levels of FSH and LH, yet their progesterone has flat-lined at an extremely low value throughout the entire cycle, especially during the days it should be at its peak. A woman's testosterone can quantify at significantly high levels while her FSH and LH remain normal, yet she does not conceive while actively trying to get pregnant. Displaying many of the signs of menopause, a perimenopausal woman who continues to cycle regularly can register normal FSH and LH. Conversely, an elevated FSH does not always indicate low estrogen.

Salivary hormone panels, on the other hand, can be expanded to include the FSH and LH, measuring the tissue concentration of the bioactive hormone fraction. A salivary analysis, therefore, allows a more precise picture when comparing the FSH with ovarian estrogen levels and the LH with progesterone levels.

SALIVA TESTING

For the woman continuing to have periods, the salivary test enables the measurement of hormones throughout an entire cycle. In the salivary hormone panel you collect your samples conveniently at home, and send them to the laboratory. The test maps the bioactive fractions of 17 beta-estradiol and progesterone as they vary throughout your cycle and includes a free testosterone level, reflecting the average of the follicular, ovulatory, and luteal phases of your cycle and your DHEA level. This approach gives numerical values for each hormone throughout one entire cycle and plots a graph showing how the estrogen and progesterone levels are fluctuating, which may be dominant or deficient, and what days during the month there is an imbalance in the ratio between them. When, or if, ovulation occurs can clearly be seen on the graph. There is a general hormonal pattern common to all cycling women, within a few days' variable. The saliva test shows if your cycle is within that normal range, and if not, it shows which hormone and when in your cycle it is out of balance. This monthlong hormone panel, with saliva samples collected on specific days, or a twenty-four-hour urine sample, collected midcycle and around day nineteen or twenty, is valuable in assessing

- PMS
- Irregular cycles prior to menopause
- Painful periods (dysmenorrhea)
- Absent cycles, as in amenorrhea
- Early ovulation
- Double ovulation
- Functional infertility
- Pregnancy problems
- Miscarriages
- Cyclic acne
- Recurrent ovarian cysts, overt and polycystic ovarian disease
- Hypothalamic-pituitary-ovarian axis disregulation
- Endometriosis
- Estrogen to progesterone imbalance
- Uterine fibroids
- Cyclic headaches and migraines
- Unusually heavy periods
- Bleeding between periods
- Loss of libido
- Excessive unwanted hair growth, as in testosterone-dependent hirsutism
- Sexual differentiation problems

Separate samples of salivary testing can also assess these problems:

- Thyroid functions—underactive (hypo) and overactive (hyper)
- Adrenal stress markers, especially to evaluate adrenal functioning, along with cortisol levels

The single sample collection, short-panel saliva test quantifies estrone, estradiol, estriol, progesterone, testosterone, and DHEA but does not indicate fluctuations throughout the month. The long panel requires two samples of saliva, usually collected about one week apart, and provides a baseline of your hormone levels with either a challenge to evaluate your response to your natural hormone therapy or to see the degree to which your hormones fluctuate on their own, independent of menstruation. Both of these tests are valuable for the perimenopausal woman who has missed several periods, and for the postmenopausal woman who has not had a cycle in over a year.

URINE TESTING

The same methodology used to test steroid levels in professional athletes is now available to access your E1, E2, E3, testosterone, DHEA, and the metabolite of progesterone. This test requires a twenty-four-hour collection of urine by you at home that is then sent to the lab. The efficacy surpasses blood analysis, especially for women currently taking any phytogenic hormones in cream form. For an accurate salivary analysis, a woman may choose to desist from taking her transdermal hormone formula to truly measure her own hormonal values. With the twenty-four-hour urine analysis, she can remain on her formula and still assess her hormonal status. Resource laboratories are listed at the end in Part Four.

UNDERSTANDING YOUR HORMONES

Balanced hormones help us to feel better and look our best, and they protect our bones and prevent Alzheimer's disease. And because we live in an era of multistressors, it is also important to sustain a healthy immune system by maintaining hormonal balance. Which hormone does what? Let's take a closer look at the primary hormones that can be accessed phytogenically and compounded—progesterone, estrogen, DHEA, and testosterone—and their role in our lives as women.

WHAT IS PROGESTERONE?

Produced by your ovaries each month while you are menstruating, with a smaller amount produced by your adrenal glands, progesterone is the most significant female reproductive hormone, especially during the last two weeks of your cycle. The corpus luteum of your ovary manufactures progesterone beginning just before ovulation and increasing rapidly after ovulation. As progesterone levels rise, estrogen levels decline.

The drop in progesterone, at the end of our cycle, causes a woman to bleed within forty-eight hours and begin a new cycle. If conception has occurred, progesterone enables the fertilized egg to become and remain viable throughout fetal development until the birth of the baby.

During our cycling years, if we experience an anovulatory cycle—that is, a cycle during which we fail to ovulate—our ovaries do not produce progesterone for that month. And when we go through menopause and cease to ovulate altogether, our ovaries no longer create progesterone at all.

Progesterone functions directly influence many of our systems. Progesterone

- Acts as a natural antidepressant
- Helps to sustain our libido
- Assists in the conversion of fat to energy
- Acts as a natural diuretic
- Regulates blood clotting
- Helps to stabilize blood sugar levels
- Assists in the production of nerve myelin
- Guards against fibrocystic breasts
- Helps defend against breast cancer
- Helps protect against endometrial cancer
- Sustains the promotion of endometrial secretions
- Aids thyroid hormone function
- Is essential for the survival of an embryo and unborn baby throughout gestation
- Assists in maintaining the proper oxygen levels of cells
- Stabilizes zinc and copper levels
- Incites bone building, osteoblasts
- Is the foundation for cortisone production as a precursor in the adrenal cortex

WHAT IS ESTROGEN?

Another job for our ovaries is to make the steroid hormone estrogen, which is responsible for the normal maturation and development of our female reproductive system and secondary sex characteristics. Women have estrogen receptors, which serve as points of attachment and communication for the hormone, in our breasts, genitals, heart, bones, brain, skin, and over three hundred different tissues.

Estrogen production normally dominates the first half of a woman's cycle, through the peak of ovulation. After ovulation occurs, estrogen rapidly declines as our progesterone rises. Each of the three estrogens— estrone (E1), estradiol (E2), and estriol (E3)—affect our systems in varied degrees. Estradiol, the primary estrogen secreted by our ovaries, stimulates our breasts the most. Estriol, which is secreted by our ovaries in small amounts and converted by our liver from estrone, exerts the greatest influence on our vagina, cervix, and vulva. In a pregnant woman, the placenta secretes large amounts of estriol. Estrone, an estrogen converted from androstenedione, formed in the ovary and by the adrenal cortex, is thought, though not proven, to be more carcinogenic.

According to Chinese medicine, estrogen as a steroid hormone falls into the category of Essence (*jing*), though not all Essence is estrogenic. When we sustain an abundant amount of Essence, we resist disease and adapt to life's changes optimally. This description of Essence, according to Chinese medicine, can clearly be applied to the *essence* of our delicate hormonal balance.

As with progesterone, estrogen is essential for specific aspects of our health. Estrogen

- Sustains the integrity and health of our skin and blood vessels
- Helps the uterus maintain tone and flexibility
- Creates the rapid reproduction of the endometrium
- Helps maintain the integrity of the urinary tract
- Initiates the adolescent growth spurt
- Starts the development and continued stimulation of breasts
- Initiates the growth of pubic and armpit hairs
- Contributes indirectly to the health of bone tissue by opposing hormones that cause calcium depletion
- Influences brain function
- Acts as the neuromodulators of memory and emotions
- Influences platelet aggregation
- Alters the lipid concentration
- Increases body fat, as stored in fat cells
- Helps prevent the oxidation of cholesterol

WHAT IS DHEA?

Dehydroepiandrosterone, commonly known as DHEA, is a product of metabolism via the steroid passageway between cholesterol and our sex steroids. Our adrenal glands provide the most abundant source of DHEA and secrete greater quantities of DHEA than of any other adrenal steroid. DHEAS, the sulfated derivative, is synthesized primarily in the liver and adrenal tissue. (Our ovaries secrete DHEA in less significant levels.) Because DHEA can convert to other hormones, including estrogen and testosterone, it has been called the "master hormone," or the "mother of all hormones." The negative aspect of this is if DHEA converts to too much testosterone, it then promotes acne and facial hair. If DHEA coverts to too much estrogen, uterine fibroids may grow, endometriosis may worsen, and women may experience an increase in the frequency of menses.

DHEA increases during pregnancy to a high level just before birth and drops at the birth. It rises to its maximum around our early twenties and then gradually declines as we age. This age-related decline does not happen with any other adrenal steroid, which suggests that perhaps some of the manifestations of aging may be due to a DHEA deficiency. The studies to date demonstrate inconclusive evidence on the relationship between DHEA levels and disease risks. However, a deficiency of DHEA is found in almost every major category of disease. This evidence suggests that DHEA may be associated with autoimmune diseases such as lupus, rheumatoid arthritis, multiple sclerosis, chronic fatigue syndrome, AIDS, allergies, osteoporosis, and Alzheimer's disease, as well as obesity, high blood pressure, and heart disease.

Although we continue to learn about DHEA functioning, some studies currently suggest that DHEA

- Prevents obesity
- Prevents diabetes
- Helps prevent cancers
- Helps prevent heart disease
- Enhances the functioning of our immune system
- Promotes antiaging factors
- Helps guard against osteoporosis
- Improves cognition and behavior in dementia and Alzheimer's disease

- Helps maintain a general sense of well-being and mood
- Acts as a building block for androgenic sex hormones

WHAT IS TESTOSTERONE?

Although we usually think of testosterone as a male hormone produced by the testes at a rate twenty times greater than that found in women, testosterone is in reality a steroid produced by our ovaries and adrenal glands as well. Testosterone is also synthesized from androstenedione, a product of DHEA and progesterone. Women have receptors for testosterone in our nipples, clitoris, and vagina, enhancing sensitivity to sexual stimulation and pleasure. Both testosterone and estrogen are transported on the same protein in our bloodstream, the sex hormone binding globulin (SHBG).

Like the other hormones we have explored, testosterone declines as we age. Many women experience a variety of physical and some emotional symptoms when their testosterone levels drop too low. Testosterone deficiency in women manifests itself as the loss of libido or sexual desire, impaired sexual function sometimes approaching repulsion or complete aversion to sex, loss of a sense of well-being, and loss of bone mass, muscle tone, and muscle strength.

Testosterone

- Enhances proper musculoskeletal development
- Helps maintain efficient functioning of cells throughout our body
- Is important in the development of the embryo by signaling the cells of a male embryo to develop as a male
- Helps maintain healthy functioning of most of the tissue in our body
- Helps sustain our sense of well-being and vital energy
- Stimulates armpit and pubic hair growth
- Stimulates the skin to produce more oil, which gives shine to hair and a healthy glow to our skin, unless it becomes an excess and produces acne in specific areas
- Enhances anabolic activity
- Enhances and sustains libido
- Enhances aerobic metabolism
- Increases protein synthesis

WHAT IS THYROID FUNCTION?

Although the thyroid hormone cannot be compounded from a phytogenic source, natural thyroid derived from a homeopathic, bovine (cow), or porcine (pig) source is available. And because symptoms of thyroid dysfunction mimic those of a progesterone deficiency, I am including it here. When our thyroid becomes dysfunctional, it becomes either underactive (hypothyroidism) or overactive (hyperthyroidism). Common and far too frequently undiagnosed, thyroid dysfunction presents a significant health problem for women.

Situated in the front of your neck, your thyroid gland consists of two halves, or lobes, that occupy the space along the windpipe (the trachea) and are connected with a narrow band of thyroid tissue called the isthmus. The function of the thyroid gland is to take iodine and convert it into thyroxine (T4) and triiodothyronine (T3), both thyroid hormones. Thyroid stimulating hormone (TSH), produced by the pituitary gland, responds to decreased levels of T3 and T4, and stimulates the thyroid gland to produce more hormones. The hypothalamus, part of our brain, regulates the pituitary gland. There are different types of thyroid receptors present in other areas of our body, which the pituitary receptors may not always interpret to be low in thyroid hormone. This might account for a normal TSH when the thyroid hormones are actually low.

Unfortunately, the routine approach to thyroid testing has been to run a serum TSH. This is inadequate to effectively evaluate a truly malfunctioning thyroid because countless levels of TSH measure within normal limits. And unless specifically requested by the practitioner who orders the test, labs typically only test the remaining thyroid functions if the TSH exhibits an abnormal value. If investigated further, a woman who presents symptoms of a thyroid problem, for example, may show her T3 or T4 to measure quite low even in the presence of a normal TSH. It seems that normal amounts of thyroid hormones are present in the bloodstream, but the cells have not received adequate T3 and T4 to function optimally.

The thyroid salivary analysis tests all the thyroid functions and at a significantly lower cost than the serum tests. Other thyroid tests include: serum T4 and T3 by RIA, a laboratory standard method; thyroid-binding globulin (TBG), an iodine uptake scan that requires that you take radioactive iodine on an empty stomach and have your thyroid scanned; thyroid ultrasound; thyroid antibody test; and thyroid needle biopsy.

Do you tend to feel cold, fatigued, irritable, and find handfuls of your hair decorating the floor much of the time? Get an oral basal body thermometer, which measures your temperature in 0.1°F increments. Once you are in bed but before you go to sleep, shake the thermometer down to its lowest point and place it within easy reach. Take your body temperature— by placing the thermometer under your tongue for ten minutes—first thing in the morning before you get out of bed and three or four times throughout the day. Do this for three to six consecutive days, noting your temperature each time on the chart on page 32. Do not do this during ovulation, the midcycle phase of your menstrual cycle. Calculate the average reading to assess the possibility of thyroid dysfunction. (Normal body temperatures are 98.6°F [Fahrenheit]/36°C [Celsius] when taken orally, about 97.6°F/35.2°C when taken under the arm, and approximately 99.6°F/37.2°C, or 0.5 to 1.0°F higher than the oral if taken rectally.) What is your average temperature? Does it repeatedly register 97.8°F or lower? This reading strongly suggests evidence of an underactive thyroid (hypothyroid).

If you are a cycling woman, just prior to ovulation your basal temperature will drop, followed by a sharp rise and immediate fall after ovulation. You want to take your temperature during the period least affected by your hormonal fluctuations, which is most stable between day two and day five of your menstrual cycle. When you make love, have a restless night, have an allergy attack, or are ill, your basal temperature will be affected, altering its accuracy for the purpose of evaluating your thyroid function.

Thyroid function

- Affects onset of menstruation (menarche) in puberty
- Supports the immune function
- Regulates menstrual flow
- Affects regularity of menses
- Prevents PMS
- Helps to prevent menstrual cramps (dysmenorrhea)
- Helps to promote optimum fertility

- Helps to prevent miscarriage
- Regulates body temperature
- Affects levels of energy and fatigue
- Affects skin, e.g., temperature, sweating, dryness, pallor; coarseness of hair; thickness of tongue
- Affects integrity of the speed of speech
- Helps to prevent depression

Common conditions associated with thyroid dysfunction, which can also suggest other possible causes, include:

With Hypothyroidism

- Acid indigestion or unexplained nausea, repeatedly, not singular or rare occurrences
- Acne, independent of age—consider dietary causes first
- Anxiety, ongoing and often out of proportion to external factors
- Asthma—consider environmental causes
- Bruise easily, independent of anemia
- Brittle or peeling finger- or toenails—also consider calcium deficiencies
- Constipation—consider dietary causes, inadequate exercise, or insufficient water intake
- Depression, similar to that experienced in PMS
- Dry eyes and eye sockets—consider your computer time
- Dry hair, independent of climate responses
- Dry skin—can also be hormonal or reflect inadequate intake of oil in your diet
- Fatigue, sustained and bordering on being chronic
- Feelings of hopelessness or lack of motivation
- Fluid retention, usually in lower half of your body and independent of diet and exercise
- Frequent infections, including unusual increased susceptibility
- Hair loss, noticeable continuous increase in hair falling out in your hands, comb, or brush (a common complaint)
- Headaches/migraines, at any time in your cycle
- High cholesterol—eliminate dietary causes
- Hives, without prior history
- Infertility, when other causes have been eliminated

- Insomnia—has many possible causes; hormonal imbalances, stress, and dietary sources most common
- Irregular, prolonged, and/or painful menses—also suggests progesterone deficiencies
- Irritability, often unexplained, with or without PMS
- Lack of concentration and inability to focus with your usual duration of attentiveness
- Libido, decrease or loss—can also be hormonal
- Low blood sugar tendency—eliminate dietary causes
- Low blood pressure, feeling faint upon rising
- Memory loss or poor memory when previously focused
- Panic attacks
- PMS, emotional or physical symptoms, refer to list in Chapter 3 (pages 47–49)
- Psoriasis, newly developed without prior history
- Tinnitus, may be experienced as a strange whooshing sound or actual ringing in the ears
- Ulcers
- Weight gain with the inability to lose excess weight

With Hyperthyroidism

- Aversion to heat, so much so that it produces agitation
- Diarrhea unexplained by diet, the presence of parasites, or other disease
- Exophthalmos, abnormal protrusion of the eyeballs in which too much of the whites are apparent
- Irritable bowel syndrome
- Nervousness and feeling jumpy, as if you want to get out of your own body
- Sweating independent of climate—consider hormonal imbalances
- Tremors, uncontrollable and noticeable vibrations of the hands

WHAT IS ADRENAL FUNCTION?

Again, although adrenal medicines are not phytogenic in nature, and consist primarily of animal glandular extracts, as you will see, it is important to include them in our discussion because of the impact of their interaction with and effect on other hormones. The adrenal glands, two

DAY	1	1	1	2	2	2	2	2	3	3	3	3	4	4	4	4	5	5	5	5	6	6	6	6
TIME																								
.5																								
.4																								
.3																								
.2																								
.1																								
99.0																								
.9																								
.8																								
.7																								
.6																								
.5																								
.4																								
.3																								
.2																								
.1																								
98.0																								
.9																								
.8																								
.7																								
.6																								
.5																								
.4																								
.3																								
.2																								
.1																								
97.0																								
.9																								
.8																								
.7																								
.6																								
.5																								
.4																								
.3																								

triangular organs resting atop our kidneys, consist of two sections. The outer portion, the cortex, produces cortisone; the center portion, the medulla, secretes adrenaline. The adrenal cortex assists in maintaining our salt and water balance, helps metabolize carbohydrates, and adjusts blood sugar. When we are under stress, the adrenal medulla produces adrenaline, the hormone epinephrine, which enhances the hyperalert status. Sustained over an extended period, this heightened state of adrenaline results in adrenal exhaustion.

Adrenal exhaustion should not be confused with either primary adrenal insufficiency, known as Addison's disease, which is caused by direct damage to the gland, or secondary, which may be due to pituitary disease or various other etiologies. Early symptoms of adrenal insufficiency involve a decrease in blood pressure, weakness, and fatigue.

Adrenal function

- Affects stability in energy levels
- Maintains physical and emotional stamina
- Affects stability of body temperature
- Supports heart and blood pressure
- Helps prevent PMS
- Affects integrity of bone density, joints, and muscles
- Affects stability of glucose regulation and digestive processes
- Supports the immune system
- Supports the nervous system
- Helps prevent depression and emotional roller-coaster rides
- Helps maintain skin integrity, turgor, and texture
- Affects stability of optimal body weight
- Helps regulate menses
- Helps prevent miscarriages
- Helps prevent dysmenorrhea

Common conditions associated with adrenal gland dysfunction can also suggest other possible causes:

Symptoms of Adrenal Exhaustion
Acne, worse with menses
Alcohol intolerance

Allergies

Alternating diarrhea and constipation

Apprehensiveness

Chronic illness

Chronic inflammation

Depression

Difficulty building muscle

Difficulty conceiving

Difficulty gaining weight

Dizziness when standing

Dry, thin skin

Dysmenorrhea

Easily gains weight

Excessive or weak appetite

Fatigue

Feeling tired much of the time

Fluid retention

Frequent menses

Hair loss

Headaches

Heart palpitations

High coffee/caffeine consumption

Hot flashes in menopause

Hypoglycemia

Inability to concentrate

Indigestion

Insomnia

Intolerance to heat or cold

Irritability

Less perspiration

Lightheadedness

Low blood pressure

Low body temperature

Menstrual irregularities

Miscarriages

Moments of confusion

Morning sickness in pregnancy

Muscle and joint pain and/or fatigue

Nervousness

Osteoporosis

Painful breasts with menses

PMS

Poor memory

Salt/sugar/sweet cravings

Skin discolorations

Skipped menses

Weakness

WHICH HORMONES ARE OUT OF BALANCE?

The Hormonal Checklist (see page 41) is a tool to help you keep track of specific symptoms as you experience them throughout your cycle. Each symptom correlates with a specific hormone. You can use this checklist as a tool to see where your hormones may need better support to reestablish your balance. Tracking symptoms over time has helped me understand where I need to make changes in hormonal formulas, and clearly demonstrates on paper the positive changes evoked by taking a phytogenic hormone formula to balance hormones.

To better understand which hormone causes each specific symptom, and to enable you to use the chart to evaluate your own hormonal status, I have listed the symptoms, along with their corresponding number from the chart, under the hormone with which the imbalance correlates.

IS IT MY PROGESTERONE?

Symptoms experienced between midcycle and into the onset of your menstrual cycle that suggest a *progesterone* deficiency include:

2. irregular cycles—either prolonged or too short, breakthrough bleeding or spotting
3. cramping
6. pelvic pain
7. breast pain
9. headaches
10. migraines
11. fainting spells

13. night sweats just before menses
14. irritability
16. crying, sometimes for no apparent reason
18. feeling clumsy or lacking motor coordination
19. increased anxiety
20. depression
21. lethargy
22. insomnia
23. feeling withdrawn
24. mood swings
25. feelings of hostility
26. nervous tension
27. feeling shaky
28. angry outbursts
29. feeling aggressive
30. mental confusion
31. feeling abusive toward yourself
32. heart racing
33. lack of libido
34. backache
35. neck pain
37. muscle and joint pain
38. joint swelling
39. weight gain
40. craving specific foods, especially chocolate or sweets
42. digestive disturbances
43. abdominal bloating
45. acne, below your mouth and/or on your cheeks
47. nausea
48. vomiting
49. increased or unusual flatulence (farting)
53. fluid retention before or with your period
54. frequent urination
55. urinary incontinence

Sometimes, an *excess* of estrogen or progesterone can present the same symptoms as a *deficiency* of estrogen or progesterone.

IS IT MY ESTROGEN?

Insufficient available *estrogen* can cause the following responses:

4. vaginal irritation
8. nipple pain
9. certain headaches
10. migraines
11. feeling faint
12. hot flashes
13. night sweats
15. fatigue
17. dizziness
18. clumsiness
21. lethargy
22. insomnia
26. nervous tension
27. feeling shaky
30. mental confusion
32. heart racing
33. lack of libido or loss of your sex drive
39. weight gain independent of your cycle
44. painful sex
46. skin changes—dry, itchy, or crawling sensation
50. heart palpitations and irregular heart rate or beat
51. easily distracted
52. increased or abnormal sweating
55. urinary incontinence

IS IT MY DHEA?

Anytime during our cycle and independent of having cycles altogether, low levels of *DHEA* can make us feel:

15. fatigue
20. depression
21. lethargy

24. mood swings
30. mental confusion
33. lack of libido
36. bone pain
37. joint pain
38. joint swelling
39. weight gain
50. irregular heart rate
51. easily distracted

IS IT MY TESTOSTERONE?

Symptoms of *testosterone* imbalance for women, anytime in the cycle or in the absence of cycles, include:

25. hostility
28. angry outbursts
29. feeling aggressive
33. lack of libido
37. muscle pain
39. weight gain, especially along with inability to maintain muscle tone and mass
45. acne

IS IT MY THYROID?

Indications that your *thyroid* is malfunctioning include:

1. bleeding, if irregular
3. cramping
4. vaginal irritation, candida
5. vaginal discharge, candida
9. frequent headaches
14. irritability
15. fatigue
19. anxiety
20. depression

21. lethargy
22. insomnia
24. mood swings
26. nervous tension
27. feeling shaky
30. mental confusion
32. heart racing
39. weight gain, continuous (independent of cyclic weight gain)
43. bloated abdomen
46. dry skin
47. nausea
50. irregular heart rate
51. easily distracted

Other thyroid dysfunction symptoms not included on this checklist include: sudden and sustained increase in hair loss, change in the texture of hair to coarse, constipation, repeated respiratory infections, weakness, slowed or even slurred speech, bulging eyes, edema of the eyelids, sudden weight loss, and skin pallor.

IS IT MY ADRENALS?

Symptoms of stressed *adrenals* or adrenal exhaustion at any time of your cycle include:

2. spotting between menses
3. cramping with menses
7. breast pain with menses
9. headaches
10. migraines
11. feeling faint
12. hot flashes
13. night sweats
14. irritability
15. fatigue
16. crying, especially when out of context or unprovoked
17. dizziness, especially upon standing

19. anxiety and apprehensiveness

20. depression

21. lethargy

22. insomnia

24. mood swings with PMS

27. feeling shaky, especially before eating or with fasting

30. mental confusion

32. heart racing and palpitations

37. muscle and/or joint pain

39. weight gain, independent of poor eating habits—can be weight loss

40. food cravings, especially salt, sugar, or sweets

41. increased appetite—also decreased appetite

42. upset stomach and indigestion

45. acne, worse before or during menses

46. dry skin and thinning of skin

53. fluid retention

Other symptoms suggestive of, but not limited to, adrenal dysfunctions include: difficulty building muscle, increased caffeine cravings, alcohol intolerance, allergies, unexplained hair loss, alternating diarrhea and constipation (can also suggest intestinal parasites or other intestinal diseases), and fertility dysfunctions.

HORMONAL CHECKLIST

DAY	DATE	MONTH 1	DATE	MONTH 2	DATE	MONTH 3
1						
2						
3						
4						
5						
6						
7						
8						
9						
10						
11						
12						
13						
14						
15						
16						
17						
18						
19						
20						
21						
22						
23						
24						
25						
26						
27						
28						
29						
30						
31						

1. bleeding
2. spotting
3. cramps
4. vaginal irritation
5. vaginal discharge
6. pelvic pain
7. breast pain
8. nipple pain
9. headaches
10. migraines
11. feeling faint

12. hot flashes
13. night sweats
14. irritability
15. fatigue
16. crying
17. dizziness
18. clumsiness
19. anxiety
20. depression
21. lethargy
22. insomnia

23. withdrawn
24. mood swings
25. hostility
26. nervous tension
27. feeling shaky
28. angry outbursts
29. feeling aggressive
30. mental confusion
31. self-abusiveness
32. heart racing
33. lack of libido

34. backaches
35. neck pain
36. bone pain
37. muscle/joint pain
38. joint swelling
39. weight gain
40. food craving
41. increased appetite
42. upset stomach
43. bloated abdomen
44. painful sex

45. acne
46. dry skin
47. nausea
48. vomiting
49. flatulence
50. irregular heart rate
51. easily distracted
52. abnormal sweating
53. fluid retention
54. frequent urination
55. urinary incontinence

NOTE: IF YOU ARE STARTING A NEW PRESCRIPTION, CIRCLE THE DAY YOU BEGIN. DAY 1 IS EITHER THE FIRST DAY OF YOUR MENSTRUAL CYCLE OR THE CALENDAR DAY IF YOU NO LONGER HAVE BLEEDING CYCLES.

PART TWO

THE HORMONE
ROLLER-COASTER RIDE

3

THE PMS CONUNDRUM

WHAT IS PMS?

Premenstrual syndrome, the term that evolved from the efforts of Drs. Katherine Dalton and Raymond Greene in 1953, is the most common disorder of the female endocrine system. PMS, a multifaceted, complex syndrome with varied symptoms, often debilitating, afflicts countless numbers of women who suffer repeatedly month after month. Symptoms usually start at the beginning of ovulation or any time after ovulation has occurred. For most women who suffer with PMS, their symptoms resolve with the onset of bleeding, though some women continue to be affected into the first day or two of their cycle. For women who refer to their menstrual cycle as their moon, PMS translates as pre-moon suffering.

As you read the lists of PMS symptoms, check to see if any of these echo your own monthly experience. Keep in mind that not every woman repeats the exact same variation of PMS each month. She can even have a PMS-free cycle during which, for some unknown reason, her own hormones spontaneously come into balance, though it may be only temporary. Many women struggle to function during this time of the month, and barely get through the day and their work. The despair many women experience will send them either to their doctor for a prescription of Prozac or to the neighborhood store for a bottle of their favorite spirits. As you will see in the following stories, the emotional and physical component of women's experience with PMS disturbed the quality of their lives and interfered with their most important relationships.

A note to help you understand the terminology of our menstrual cycle, also known as period, menses, moon, or moon cycle: Day one of your cycle is the first day you begin bleeding. If you experience a little spotting the day before, you still count the day of actual bleeding as day one. The length of your cycle is defined as from day one of this bleeding to the first day of the next time you bleed. A regular cycle is what is regular for you. If every month there are twenty-eight days from the first day of one period until the first day of the next, you have a twenty-eight-day cycle. The same is true if your pattern follows thirty or forty days. Pattern is the key to the term *regular cycle*. An irregular cycle is when you bleed unpredictably—for example, one month your menses may occur on the twenty-fifth day, and the next cycle may not come for fifty days, followed by another period three weeks later.

Ovulation, the ripening and rupture of the mature follicle with the release of the egg, or ovum, from your ovary, usually, but not always, transpires in the middle of your cycle. Ovulation happens on day fourteen in the average twenty-eight-day cycle.

PMS SYMPTOMS THAT RESOLVE WITH PROGESTERONE THERAPY

I have separated these PMS symptoms into two primary categories: psychological/emotional and physical. It is possible to have any combination of these responses to an insufficient progesterone production or actual progesterone deficiency. Although the manifestation of each symptom, physical or emotional, is dramatically different, compounded phytogenic progesterone effectively resolves both categories.

Progesterone therapy stimulates a woman's hormonal production of progesterone to reestablish the internal balance needed to feel anchored into your sense of who you are every day, not just certain days of the month. I have heard many women express how they feel "normal" during the first part of their cycle. Then sometime around the middle of their cycle this stranger begins to take over and control how they feel, what they say, and how they react in any given scenario, regardless of whether it is stressful or not. Even if the symptoms remain only physical, the changes feel dramatic and often disturbing or incapacitating.

Nineteen Psychological and Emotional Symptoms

1. Excessive use of alcohol, drugs, or other escape mechanisms
2. Crying or weeping spontaneously, which may be uncontrollable and either exaggerated for the circumstance, inappropriate, or unprovoked
3. Feelings of panic, usually without warning and beyond one's control to change
4. Easily frustrated and having a very short fuse
5. Feeling violent, aggressive, or hostile
6. Feeling self-abusive or actually inflicting injury upon yourself
7. Sudden anger and angry outbursts, with greater intensity than a situation may deserve, or that may be completely unprovoked by any known external cause
8. Feelings of anxiety, often unexplained or irrational
9. Verbal and/or physical abuse directed at those you love most: children, parents, lover, husband, best friend
10. Inability to focus or concentrate
11. Irritability
12. Mental exhaustion
13. Depression
14. Feelings of hopelessness
15. Mood swings
16. Feelings of being crazy
17. Attempted suicide
18. Feeling withdrawn
19. Feeling hysterical or actual hysteria

These emotional symptoms, in combination or singly noted, alter one's perception of the self and everything else in one's reality. To what extreme these symptoms are expressed remains relative to the degree of progesterone deficiency. When symptoms begin depends upon the actual day in a woman's cycle that progesterone begins to decline, and how rapidly or insufficiently it rises. This can be as early as day twelve in a twenty-eight-day cycle, or day nine in a twenty-one-day cycle.

Forty-two Physical Symptoms

1. Headaches, migraines
2. Decreased motor coordination

3. Lethargy
4. Physical exhaustion
5. Insomnia
6. Sleep disturbances
7. Night sweats
8. Interference with dream recall
9. Muscle cramps
10. Low backache
11. Gallbladder symptoms
12. Frequent urination
13. Hypoglycemic reactions
14. Food cravings
15. Increased appetite
16. Dark circles under eyes
17. Joint and muscle pain
18. Increased hair loss
19. Acne
20. Infertility
21. Breast engorgement
22. Breast tenderness/pain
23. Cold extremities
24. Being accident prone
25. Clumsiness
26. Increased sex drive
27. Lowered or lost sex drive
28. Dizziness
29. Abdominal bloating
30. Weight gain
31. Fluid retention, edema
32. Constipation/diarrhea
33. Candidiasis
34. Increased flatulence
35. Slow digestion
36. Lack of appetite
37. Puffy eyes
38. Facial pallor
39. Flare-up of arthritis

40. Greasy hair
41. Dry hair
42. Dry or oily skin

WEEPING WILL-O'-THE-WISP COMPETES WITH THE RAGING WITCH

Wild mood swings, depression, loss of a vital sense of well-being send some women to the psychiatrist's couch and add great wealth to the coffers of pharmaceutical companies. Previously, women were committed to institutions. Although taking antidepressants or anitanxiety drugs can offer temporary relief, these drugs have side effects and do not correct the underlying cause if it is rooted in a hormonal imbalance, most commonly a progesterone insufficiency or deficiency.

At a dinner party, I met one of the local psychiatrists for the first time. As I introduced myself, his mouth unabashedly dropped open, his eyes widened. He repeated my name aloud a couple of times, almost in a muttering-to-himself fashion. I began to wonder if he had had too much wine. But he recovered from his apparent shock and said, "So *you're* the one I've been bad-mouthing all these years. I must apologize. You see, treating mental or emotional problems with drug therapy is the way I was trained. I thought your approach, using these plant-based hormones, was, quite frankly, ludicrous, until I saw improvement in some women patients we share. Some of them weaned themselves off the antidepressants I prescribed and continue to take your hormones."

He shook his head and laughed.

Pamela's experience, age thirty-six
Pamela, a thirty-six-year-old mother of two, and potentially soon to be divorced, felt desperate. Her degree of PMS expressed itself with intense, uncontrollable anger, and she directed this anger with daggers at her husband. They had separated when she first came in.

> *I don't know what's wrong with me. Normally I'm a relatively calm, rational woman. It's not like me to yell at people, especially those I love. It's getting worse and I'm getting scared that I'm losing myself.*

After Pamela's tears stopped, I asked when she first noticed this change. Was there any pattern to it? Had she noticed when in her cycle her rational self took a holiday?

> *My husband could tell you exactly when I turn into Mrs. Hyde. But he's taking a holiday from me. It's really hard on the kids. I don't want to take it out on them . . . that's why I'm so scared. I threw a plate at the wall and smashed it. My moon started the next day and I started feeling more like me again. Actually, now that you mention it, Harry, my husband, would say things like "You must be getting your period, hon" every time I ragged at him. Then . . . it just seemed to fuel my fire. He would just really piss me off. When I attacked him—I actually hit him—he left. I don't think I've been quite right since little Harry was born six years ago.*

For Pamela and her family, her PMS was so severe it became a living nightmare. She became a woman out of control, screaming at her husband, breaking things, and physically lashing out. When she monitored the change in her behavior, she noticed it crept up on her beginning with ovulation, somewhere around day fourteen of her cycle. The closer she got to her period, the shorter her fuse became and the more frequent the incidents of angry outbursts.

Three months after taking 100 mg of progesterone twice a day from day twelve through day twenty-eight, she returned to discuss any changes in how she felt.

> *Harry is moving back in. We've been spending time together, even right before my moon. At first he was skeptical. He didn't see how smearing on a cream could make any difference in this crazy woman who was his wife. I have been keeping track of my cycle and how I feel. The first month I felt less edgy; by the end of the second, I caught myself smiling and laughing and just feeling more like me. When my moon time came, it surprised me because I felt so good. I think this is working.*

Pamela suffered from progesterone insufficiency. Her pregnancy had disturbed her hormonal balance. As we explored further, she recalled the first couple of months after giving birth:

It seems a bit of a blur, though I remember crying most of the time. But I don't remember why I cried so much. I was happy to have the baby. So was Harry. It didn't make any sense that I felt depressed. I think it started around the third day after little Harry was born. I remember taking a soiled diaper to the laundry room. The next thing I knew, I was sitting on the stairs crying hysterically. It went on for some time and eventually I just made myself get a grip, get over it, and get it together. The doctor offered me an antidepressant. But I didn't want to stop nursing my baby, which I would have had to do because of the side effects and because the drug gets into breast milk.

Like many women, Pamela experienced a severe decline in her progesterone levels by the end of her pregnancy. Through utter willpower she compensated for this deficiency. But her hormonal balance did not begin to recover until she supplemented with progesterone. She continued taking the progesterone consistently for six months. She felt so much improvement that she decided to discontinue through one cycle to see how she would do on her own. After she had not taken any progesterone for six weeks, we tested her progesterone level. It was within the normal range for that phase of her cycle. She and Harry were about to take their first vacation together in many years, without any children, a second honeymoon. Pamela felt a little nervous, but excited. "I'm taking my cream with me, just in case," she told me.

In hindsight, Pamela would have benefited significantly from the use of progesterone after she had given birth, and perhaps during her pregnancy as well. After consulting your physician, you may want to use progesterone during or shortly following your pregnancy. "There have been no adverse effects on fetal development reported when natural progesterone is used during pregnancy," says Neils H. Lauersen, M.D., of Mount Sinai Medical Center in New York, the author of *Premenstrual Syndrome and You.* On the other hand, synthetic progestin can adversely affect the developing fetus.

Rachel's experience, age twenty-three
Several years ago I received a call from Rachel's boyfriend, Tom. As he spoke, I could hear his concern for Rachel, as well as his fears.

Can you talk to her? We've been getting along great, communicating well, our sex life is excellent, better than ever. But suddenly she went off on me, couldn't even tell me why. Rachel just went into a fit of rage, screaming at me. I can't remember exactly what I said to her that set her off. But she lost it. I think I asked her if she wanted to go to the market with me. Can I put her on right now, please?

In the background, as I waited, I could hear Tom's compassionate and gentle approach to bring Rachel, racked with tears, to the phone. After several belly-wrenching sobs, and after catching her breath, Rachel spoke.

This doesn't make any sense. Things have been going well. Something inside me snapped and I don't remember what happened next.

When I asked her where she was in her cycle, she went blank and had a difficult time remembering when her last menstrual period had occurred. We talked about other things for a few moments and then Rachel realized it had been about two weeks earlier. She burst into tears again.

This is the first good man I've been with in a very long time. I don't want to mess this up. I don't want to lose him. But if I don't get some help immediately, he'll be out of here.

I had 100 mg progesterone capsules on hand for just this sort of weekend emergency. The local pharmacy had not yet begun to offer compounded hormones, and it would take several days to get a formula mailed to Rachel.

She came over as soon as we finished the call. Anxiously, Rachel immediately began taking the 100 mg of progesterone in an oral capsule twice a day. Two days later, Tom called to tell me that Rachel had returned to normal and to offer his gratitude for the remedy.

At twenty-three years of age, Rachel had experienced her first-known episode of PMS. She was shocked at her behavior, which apparently had been wilder than either of them had shared with me, and stunned at the intensity of the attack and her lack of self-control. Normally, Rachel prided herself on her grip on reality, her fervent degree of self-control, her ability to focus and remain rational in tense situations, until this incident.

ACNE AND PMS

Alexa's experience, age fourteen

At fourteen years of age, Alexa had lost her zest for life and developed recurring acne one week before her period. Her mother had been working on her menopausal symptoms when she began to notice a pattern in her daughter's withdrawn behavior and the acne outbreaks. The acne erupted primarily on her chin and lower cheek area. Because of the consistency in this pattern, Alexa's mother wondered if her daughter suffered from a hormonal imbalance. My first visit with Alexa was quiet. When I asked her to tell me what was going on, her first response was: "I don't know why my mom sent me here. There's nothing wrong with me." Most of that visit consisted of me asking questions and Alexa giving me monosyllabic answers or a blank look, during which she avoided eye contact. She agreed to chart her cycle for one month, and test her hormone levels.

As I suspected, her progesterone was unusually low even for a young teenager who had been menstruating for two years. She did not want to take her progesterone in capsules because she was already having trouble when she took her vitamins. The vitamins seemed to make her nauseated. Alexa opted to try progesterone in the transdermal cream form, but she could not remember to use it with any reliability. So we moved on to progesterone in sublingual drops. Beginning on day ten of her cycle until her period started, Alexa took 50 mg of progesterone, dissolved in olive oil, under her tongue in the morning and at bedtime. Three months later, she returned.

> *It's like really weird. I didn't realize what had been happening to me. I haven't had a zit in three months. My mom made sure I took my drops and I actually marked on my calendar when I was supposed to start. I think I might have forgotten a few times, you know, like when I spent the night over at a friend's house. It was too lame to take a bottle of drops with me. Do I need to keep taking them now?*

Before her visit, her mother had called to tell me what a difference the progesterone had made in Alexa. "I feel like I have my old Alexa back. She smiles more and seems more interested in doing things again." We discontinued the progesterone after three months and she has continued to do well on her own for four years. Alexa's acne and PMS were due to the instability in her progesterone.

It can take years for the hormone levels of some young women to even out after the onset of menarche, the beginning of the menstrual cycles. In Alexa's experience, once she became somewhat consistent in taking her progesterone, her own hormones were stimulated and coerced into balance. For her, as with many other teenage girls, the progesterone therapy was short term.

IRREGULAR CYCLES AND PMS

Iris's experience, age forty-four

> *I just can't go on like this. I feel like a crazy woman. This is definitely not the example of womanhood I want to set for my daughter. She'll be a teenager soon, starting her period. And I don't want to be a raving lunatic who bleeds every couple of weeks.*

At forty-four years of age, Iris, who usually had a regular twenty-one-day cycle, began to experience more frequent menses with brownish spotting starting on day seventeen. Along with the spotting to bright red bleeding with clotting, she also noticed some facial hair that came around the same time. Although she had been under more stress than usual, this did not explain her wild mood swings during which she would feel like she was in a fit of rage one minute and crying the next. A cream of 10 percent progesterone with 12.5 mg DHEA, which she applied twice a day consistently for six months, returned her cycle to a normal rhythm. When she returned in six months, she shared:

> *Oh my God, Saundra, I really thought I was going to lose it back then. I didn't recognize myself. And when I found myself shrieking at Daniela, well, to be honest, it really freaked me out. I could see this crazy woman step into me and take over. I lost complete control. Another freaky thing about it was that some part of my rational mind could watch this bizarre scenario take place, but it could do nothing to stop it. The first month I used the cream, I forgot to put it on*

sometimes. But I still noticed I felt more like myself and my period came on time. No pain with my period or ovulation. When I realized the cream actually made a difference, I made sure I used it every twelve hours, like clockwork.

After the next five months of normal, PMS-free cycles, Iris experimented with her cream whenever she felt she needed it intermittently over the next two years. Then she went off the progesterone and DHEA altogether. She sustained her own hormonal balance for the next three years. At that time, perimenopausal symptoms began to arise, which required a reassessment of her hormonal status and the introduction of estrogen into her formula.

VOMITING, PAIN, AND PHYSICAL PMS

Violette's experience, age twenty-seven

Several hours before my period starts, the pain is so intense, I double over, vomit, and then pass out. At first the nausea begins in waves and I get distracted and have trouble thinking. Next, my entire lower abdomen feels like it's caught in some sort of medieval Vise-Grip torture device. The pain is so intense my head starts to spin—no, I think it's more that the whole room is spinning. I throw up and faint. When I come back around, my head pounds, and although nothing looks right, I can't close my eyes and light makes it all much worse. So I lie curled up with the lights low and try to focus on breathing and not vomiting again. If I get enough warning, I take drugs just to get me through the day. Otherwise, the drugs make me more nauseated and I vomit more. About two weeks before I get my period, I start to feel shaky, I get heart palpitations, I gain five pounds, which seems to be mostly water retention. Oh, and my breasts swell and hurt. I feel really tired, but that's probably because I hardly sleep for those two weeks.

In addition to all of these severe and disturbing physical symptoms, at twenty-seven, Violette complained of mood swings, irritability, and anxiety attacks simultaneously. For two weeks each month, Violette functioned minimally, and she remained completely incapacitated for two days every month.

Although Violette had a regular, thirty-day cycle, her hormonal analysis clearly showed a low progesterone pattern throughout the cycle, right from the beginning with a slight rise around day twenty-four, and progressing to virtually no available progesterone just prior to the arrival of her bleeding.

As we discussed her lifestyle and eating habits, I discovered her addiction to sugar and carbohydrates, in every possible form. The first month of her treatment consisted of a major change in her diet (see the discussion of diet and PMS, page 60) and of taking progesterone, in oral capsules, every twelve hours, daily. Her first dosage—35 mg of progesterone—began on day two of her cycle and ran through day fourteen. On days fifteen, sixteen, and seventeen, she took 50 mg of progesterone, increasing to 75 mg for days eighteen through twenty-four. The dosage went up to 100 mg on days twenty-five to twenty-eight and back down to 50 mg for the remaining days before her period.

Violette observed significant improvement in that first cycle. She felt less irritable and did not experience any sensation of shakiness. Her breast tenderness and swelling was minimal, she experienced no heart palpitations, and felt less bloated. When her bleeding began, she did not vomit or faint, nor did she double over with pain. The much milder cramps seemed subdued and she only needed 400 mg of ibuprofen. However, the migraine that accompanied her cycle did not completely fade away. Although the vertigo disappeared, she still needed the lights low and a day in bed.

The next month she was armed with extra progesterone in a 10 percent cream to apply at the very first sign of a headache. The day before she expected her period, as soon as she felt the familiar pulse in her head that seemed to go along with a sense of disorientation, Violette massaged a fingerful of cream into her temples and forehead. Not wanting to risk the possibility of this developing into a migraine, she repeated her application two hours later, and again in another two hours. She also rubbed some over her entire lower abdomen.

I was so determined to see if I could have a painless cycle, I practically took a bath in the stuff. Well, I'm exaggerating. At first I didn't think the cream would prevent the headache, but it never got any worse than that initial awareness I had that it was about to start. And instead of the wild pain that doubled me over, I only felt a vague dull aching the first day. I didn't go back to bed.

This was the first *normal* cycle of her life. She had suffered from severe dysmenorrhea (painful periods) and PMS ever since her cycles began. The necessity for the additional progesterone waned within the following cycle. Although she resisted the diet that required her to decrease her refined-food intake, Violette discovered she felt better and had more energy in general when she ate smaller meals more frequently and cut down on the sugars and carbohydrates. Currently, she continues taking 100 mg of progesterone twice a day, enjoying a freedom to live her life more completely and pain-free each day of the month.

PROGESTERONE, PLEASE, AND QUICK

Whether a woman experiences primarily emotional or physical symptoms, I have found that by treating PMS with compounded natural phytogenic progesterone, we achieve resolution of the symptoms within a relatively short period. If a woman is able to begin her first dosage of progesterone early enough in her cycle, just before or around ovulation, she notices significant relief in that first cycle.

Do you experience any of the symptoms listed at the beginning of this section? Each of these symptoms, as well as their underlying causes, can be eliminated with natural progesterone therapy. I have known women who have been affected to such an extreme degree that they feel either suicidal or as though they need an exorcism before their period, month after month.

Do you notice a consistent, recurrent, cyclic pattern of not feeling like yourself? Write down how you feel during this phase of your cycle. When we write it in our own words, our minds do not play the "Well, maybe I imagined it" game. And when a similar scenario repeats itself, particularly during the same phase of your cycle, a pattern has been established.

The twenty-four-hour urine or salivary hormonal analysis, as well as your experience of the symptoms, will clarify whether this pattern results from any hormonal imbalance.

If at this time you cannot, or choose not, to evaluate your hormonal profile, yet you truly believe you experience PMS due to a progesterone deficiency, you can initiate progesterone therapy with an nonprescription 10 percent progesterone cream. Use one-quarter to one-half teaspoon every twelve hours, from midcycle until your period begins. Discontinue the progesterone and allow your period to flow, although it is safe to use it during the first day to eliminate cramps.

Keep in mind that if you decide to evaluate your hormones, and you are currently taking any cream hormonal therapeutic approach, prescription or over the counter, the results will be influenced by your formula and will not accurately reflect your hormone levels. The advantage of doing the salivary hormone analysis throughout an entire cycle is to clarify whether other hormones, in addition to progesterone, need support, and to numerically calculate the dosage of progesterone in precise amounts throughout your cycle. The analysis gives you an accurate baseline of your hormonal fluctuations and shows if you follow a normal pattern with numerical hormone values.

Progesterone, prescribed for you by your practitioner from a compounding pharmacy, is available in specified micronized dosages, ranging from 5 mg to 100 mg for each dose, to be absorbed using one of three different approaches. In an oral capsule, the progesterone is dissolved in olive or safflower oil to prevent its destruction by stomach acid when it is swallowed. In the transdermal approach, progesterone mixed into a cream with a safflower or other vegetable oil base is applied directly to your skin. This is most effectively absorbed through soft tissue—armpits, upper inner arms, chest, abdomen, inner thighs, behind your knees, buttocks, and inner labia. Make sure the cream does not contain any alcohol before applying it to your labia as one of the application sites. (Alcohol will burn fragile tissue and can increase dryness.) The third method of absorption is under your tongue, in sublingual drops, also dissolved most commonly in olive oil.

The transdermal approach interfaces least with the liver. So, for example, if you have had or currently have hepatitis or any other stress to your liver, this is the best approach. Also, if you have consistent digestive disturbances, you may not absorb as well through the gut, as in the oral capsule, and the transdermal route may yield the quickest, most effective results. When you utilize the transdermal route of administration, it is important to rotate the places where you apply the cream. Rotating locations literally means that you daily change the site where you apply the cream for each dose. For example, one day you apply the morning and evening dose to your upper inner arms, the next day use your inner thighs, and so on. We have receptors in our skin that pick up the encoded hormone information and send this information along a neural pathway to our brain, which then disperses the hormone directly into our bloodstream. When progesterone cream is repeatedly applied to the same location, our brain receives the message that we have enough progesterone and do not need to absorb more. Instantly, we lose the benefit of the hormone essential to our balance.

Many of the OTC natural progesterones have other ingredients in the cream in addition to progesterone. Some of these ingredients include Chinese herbs, phytoestrogens, aromatherapy fragrances, vitamin E, and other substances thought to be beneficial. Usually, when treating PMS, you do not want phytoestrogens in your formula. Therefore, if you want to use OTC progesterone, choose one without phytoestrogens and one that tells you the exact number of milligrams each dose contains.

WHAT ELSE HELPS PMS?

Today, the savvy woman chooses to educate herself and not merely accept her lot in life, especially when it concerns her health, well-being, and ability to function at her optimum. If you suffer from PMS, you do not have to tough this out. You do not have to be plagued by or limited by the symptoms during part of each month. PMS is not a normal state of being. And over a period of years, PMS can evolve to include other conditions reflective of low progesterone.

PMS May Develop Into
- Infertility
- Miscarriage, spontaneous abortion
- Endometriosis

- Menstrual disorders
- Ovarian cysts
- Prolonged psychological disorders
- Breast disease
- Uterine fibroids
- Perimenopausal difficulties
- Osteoporosis

I invite you to explore more options, in addition to hormones, to enhance your sense of optimal health. These next sections describe changes you can make in your diet, herbal and homeopathic remedies, nutritional supplements, sex as PMS therapy, and the balancing qualities of stress reduction, exercise, and time out for you and you alone.

PMS DIETARY ADJUSTMENTS

A diet high in protein, high in fiber, and low in sugar and carbohydrates helps in eradicating PMS symptoms. Discover how to nurture yourself without relying on comfort foods that worsen your symptoms. Honor the variations of your own rhythm. This is important regardless of your age.

When the chocolate cravings start, remember that if we crave sugar, we require protein. Actually, sugar, especially refined white sugar, significantly increases PMS symptoms. During the week or two before your period, eat smaller meals, high in protein and fiber, and eat more frequently, even if you do not have much of an appetite. The best protein sources are soybeans, whey, and fresh fish. Deep-ocean fish are the healthiest and cleanest, rather than fish caught in more polluted waters. For more information on dolphin-safe fishing, and turtle-safe shrimp, go to *www.cmc-ocean.org* and *www.wholefoodsmarket.com/issues/list-sea food.html*.

For nonvegetarians, chicken and turkey are also good sources of protein. (Beef and pork, unless it comes from free-range, organically fed, hormone-free animals, should be avoided for the same reasons that one should avoid commercially grown poultry.) Conventional poultry contains many unhealthy components that promote stress to and the potential breakdown of our immune system. Commercially grown poultry are

usually fed grain grown with pesticides and possibly genetically engi-
neered corn or other feed. Regularly administered exogenous synthetic
hormones—given to make the chicks and turkeys grow faster and fatter
than nature intends—produce a more marketable product faster. Antibiotics given to deal with or prevent infections—often caused by the
crowded, inhumane living conditions found in many large poultry
farms—contribute to an imbalance in our own internal pH, stress our
immune system, and promote the overgrowth of systemic candidiasis
and vaginal yeast infections when we consume the poultry.

When you eat this poultry on a regular basis, you are also eating the
synthetic hormones in the meat and eggs, which alter our own hormonal
balance. These exogenous hormones that you have now consumed exacerbate PMS symptoms by increasing your own estrogen hormone
levels. So, if you eat poultry and eggs, it is important to buy free-range,
pesticide-free, certified organic poultry and eggs raised without hormones and antibiotics. Red meats, although felt by many to be a good
source of protein, may, because of the high content of uric acid, also aggravate PMS symptoms.

A diet free of refined sugars, white flours, and refined cereals can help
prevent dysmenorrhea (painful menstruation), which is often exacerbated or caused by constipation. Refined, *enriched* foods containing additives and chemicals are digested more slowly and tax our systems, and
their by-products cling to the intestinal and colon walls. As these by-
products clog the colon, constipation ensues. Due to the anatomical location of your uterus—in front of the lower colon—when you are
constipated, the full bowel applies pressure to the uterus. With the onset
of menstruation, the uterine muscle contracts as it sheds the endometrial
lining. These are very mild contractions; however, against the pressures
of a full bowel, the contractions will be more painful than if there were
nothing creating resistance.

Foods to Avoid Include
- Any processed foods with additives
- White breads and pastas
- Any cereal that does not contain whole grains
- Foods and drinks high in sugar
- Alcohol

- Salty foods and snacks
- Soft drinks—the sugarless ones as well

Foods designed for dieters who wish to lose weight often contain artificial sweeteners—saccharine, sucaryl, and aspartame, also
known as NutraSweet, Equal, Spoonful, and Equal Measure, which
are significantly more harmful than regular sugar. Go to *www.nexus
magazine.com* for more information on the serious dangers of aspartame.

If you have a sweet tooth, try stevia, a South American herb that is
safe even for diabetics to use and contains no calories. Raw sugar, when
used within reasonable limits, will not increase a tendency to gain
weight. It is those refined carbohydrates we've talked about that will
cause you to gain weight. Choose, instead, natural fresh foods; they will
provide essential vitamins and minerals, nutrients the body needs for
proper digestion and assimilation to help keep you feeling balanced and
healthy.

HOMEOPATHIC REMEDIES FOR PMS

For those of you who respond to homeopathy, PMS remedies are specific to the symptoms. Homeopathy is a unique, systematic, scientific
method of therapy based on the principle of stimulating a person's own
healing process. Founded on the law of similars—that is, "like cures
like"—homeopathic remedies are derived from substances that produce
the symptoms of a disease in a healthy person. In homeopathic form,
that substance is converted, something like a vaccine is converted,
and can potentially cure a sick person. The strength or "potency" of a
homeopathic remedy is measured in terms of X, C, or M, unlike other
medicines, which are quantified in micrograms, milligrams, grams, or
international units.

- *Apis* relieves the intensity associated with almost violent downward-
  pressure pain and dark mucousy blood. Some women actually feel as
  if they're in labor when their menses begins.
- *Belladonna* helps if your flow is bright red and your pelvic pain makes
  you feel as if your entire pelvis is trying to push itself out, through a
  bearing-down sensation.

- *Chamomilla* can relieve your mood when you feel impatient and when your fuse is short, independent of excess sugar or caffeine, and it can alleviate cramps.
- *Nux Vomica* is another good remedy when we feel irritable.

These are but a few of the many homeopathic remedies that can help.

If you know your constitutional remedy, start with it to reestablish your inner balance. You may want to see a homeopathic practitioner or research homeopathic remedy pictures until you find one that fits you. Some websites with homeopathic information, some of which include on-line consultations, are *www.homeopathyhome.com/; www.homeopathic.org/; www.indiaspace.com/homeopathy/; www.elixirs.com/;* and *www.hahnemannlabs.com/.*

HERBAL PMS HELPERS

There are PMS herbal formulas aplenty at your local whole-food grocer, natural food store, and on-line herbal apothecary. If you know you respond better to Chinese herbs than Western herbs, this narrows your choices. There are several Chinese herbal formulas that assist in treating PMS symptoms.

- *Bupleurum and Tang Kuei Formula, Xiao Yao San,* produced by Golden Flower Chinese Herbs, regulates and harmonizes the energy of the liver and spleen, specifically to help with tenderness, distension, lumps, and fibrocystic tendencies in your breasts, bloating, depression, emotional instability, irritability, moodiness, fatigue, headaches, dizziness, irregular cycles, and menstrual cramps. This formula should not be used if you have abdominal distension or signs of excess heat defined by excessive vital function demonstrating feverishness, flushed face, thirst with the desire for cold drinks, constipation, a rapid pulse, and reddening of the tongue with a yellowish coating.
- When heat is present, according to Drs. John Scott and Lorena Monda, founders of Golden Flower Chinese Herbs, use *Free and Easy Wanderer Plus, Jia Wei Xiao Yao San,* instead. This formula assists with increased anxiety, angry outbursts, depression, irritability, rest-

lessness, emotional instability, as well as breast pain, swelling, and lumps; menstrual nausea and vomiting; and irregular and painful periods. Do not take this if you think you might be pregnant.

- *Tang Kuei and Peony Formula, Dang Gui Shao Yao San,* another woman's tonic, primarily focuses on balancing the physical PMS symptoms.
- *Beauty Pearl,* by Sun Rider, assists with PMS symptoms through the focus of balancing hormones.
- *Dong Quai,* taken in a tincture, 15 drops four times a day for up to seven days, can induce a late menses and temporarily relieve the edginess of PMS.
- Tea made from fresh *gingerroot* or *licorice root* soothes and relieves cramping, while the aroma relaxes your spirit.

Other Western herbs, found in tinctures, capsules, or loose for tea, can also help with PMS.

- *Black Cohosh* calms hysteria and relieves cramps.
- *Chasteberry* combats breast pain, fluid retention, headaches, and fatigue. It appears to help increase progesterone.
- *Cramp Bark* relaxes your nerves and relieves cramps and spasms.
- *Damiana,* 375 mg three times a day, acts as a diuretic, works directly on the reproductive system, and is an aphrodisiac.
- *Dandelion Root* helps with cramps and constipation.
- *Evening Primrose Oil,* a natural source of the fatty acid gamma-linolenic acid, helps relieve menstrual cramps and breast swelling, lumps, and pain.
- *Feverfew,* an anti-inflammatory herb, also stimulates the uterus.
- *Licorice Root,* containing phytoestrogenic as well as antiviral properties, alleviates cramps.
- *Oregon Grape Root,* 150 mg, helps to purify the blood; in combination with 30 mg of *Cascara Sagrada Bark,* it assists in digestion and absorption, as well as preventing constipation. However, I think *Cascara Sagrada* can be a rather harsh herb.
- *Sarsaparilla,* 500 mg a day, taken a week or two before your period, has diuretic qualities, and is useful if you suffer from fluid retention.
- Uncompounded *Wild Yam Root,* 200 mg a day, can stimulate your

body to increase your own progesterone production, but it is not as effective as compounded phytogenic progesterone.

VITAMINS, MINERALS, AND PMS

Beyond diet and various remedies, it is important to make sure you take in adequate quantities of vitamins and minerals—B-6, B-12, B complex, calcium, magnesium, zinc, iron, and vitamins A, D, E, and C—all of which continue to remain vital. This section gives an overview of the vitamins and minerals essential for women during the second half of their cycle. For more in-depth information on vitamins and minerals, explore *www.nutrition.org/nutrinfo/* or *www.itc.utk.edu/~zemel/UH338/vitsup.html.* There are literally thousands of resource sites on the Web. I found these two to have clear information with easy access.

Without isolating the function of each, in general, *B vitamins* calm the nervous system; affect some instances of depression and confusion; are necessary to assist in the metabolism of fats, proteins, carbohydrates, and amino acids; have an anti-gray-hair factor; and exhibit antianemic qualities. A balanced B complex takes the edge off PMS.

Calcium prevents muscle cramps and helps to promote blood clotting. Some women who experience PMS test deficient for calcium and magnesium. Calcium requires *magnesium, vitamin E,* and *vitamin C* for adequate absorption. *Vitamin D* increases the assimilation of calcium. *Boron* and *zinc* also assist in absorption and utilization of calcium. When mixed with the B vitamins, calcium soothes the nervous system. For PMS, increase your calcium to 1,200 mg along with at least 600 mg or an equal amount of magnesium. If you have difficulty sleeping during this phase of your cycle, take your calcium and magnesium at bedtime, separately from your other vitamins and minerals. For further augmentation of your ability to utilize your calcium supplement, add 400 units of vitamin D, 750–1,000 mg of vitamin C, 800 units of vitamin E, and 45 mg of zinc.

As hemoglobin requires *iron*, without which our red blood cells could not live, we need to maintain our iron levels, especially before menses. Women need more iron than men because we bleed each month. Blood loss can cause anemia. Women's bodies must absorb iron (ferrous compounds) as a salt, such as ferrous gluconate, carbonate, sulfate, or fumerate, along with vitamin C to aid this absorption. And since we actually *absorb* only a portion of what we consume, dosages range as high as 325 mg.

To help prevent PMS, take 800–1,000 units of *vitamin E* daily for three to five days before you expect your cycle to begin. Vitamin E, an antioxidant, protects tissue, helps with muscle repair, and effects electron transfer (when one electron leaves an element to join another element). Vitamin E is necessary to maintain each muscular system, including the uterus, and it also stimulates the production of female hormones. So, via both of these mechanisms, vitamin E helps decrease cramps and even out our hormones. Another function of vitamin E is to stimulate the thyroid. Many symptoms of hypothyroidism, an underactive thyroid dysfunction, mimic the symptoms of PMS.

One of the things *vitamin A* does is maintain the integrity of the cilia, threadlike tiny hairs in the fallopian tubes. It is these cilia that move the ovum from your ovary into your uterus. So vitamin A is as responsible for a woman's fertility as is vitamin E. It also affects the dryness and texture of our skin, including our labia, those precious lips guarding our inner gateway.

If you take each of these vitamins separately, you must swallow a handful of pills, which some find impossible to accomplish. I have heard stories out of the surgical suites in which literally handfuls of vitamins, in a hard tablet form, had caused bowel obstructions and required surgical removal. It is important to maximize your ability to break down and utilize vitamins. I find that capsules, liquids, or chewable forms are more easily digestible.

Look at *natural* vitamins, minerals, and antioxidant formulas that are designed for women, especially those that target PMS symptoms, and choose one that seems appropriate to your problems. I encourage you to trust your intuition, but do your research with different brands. Although natural vitamins and minerals tend to be more expensive, they are more effective and a healthier option. To test the efficacy of the formula you select, take it for one month. If you notice positive changes, continue taking it. A month is a reasonable length of time to evaluate the effectiveness of a product. Don't continue to invest your money in something if it fails to elicit any perceptible benefit. You're the one paying for it, and you want the benefits to be readily apparent.

SEX THERAPY FOR PMS

Does your sex drive increase along with your PMS symptoms? Or does your libido seem to evaporate altogether? Do you feel more juicy and alive as you get closer to the time you will bleed? Or do you withdraw into your private cave, feeling too frumpy to be seen by anyone, least of all your lover? Or is this the time when, for whatever reason, you make love alone?

As your hormones shift, connecting eye to eye with your lover in the face of your most genuine self, regardless of how intense your experience of PMS might be, is actually good therapy. To bare your soul and not pretend to be anything other than who you are in the moment takes courage and practice, but the rewards will astonish you. And yes, it takes an understanding partner to get close and intimate when you cry over nothing apparent one moment and burst into an angry fury the next. Yet when we communicate what we are going through to the person with whom we feel the deepest love and connection, it is truly empowering.

In those moments of raw honesty, so prevalent in the throes of any style of PMS, connecting deeply and intimately can be the greatest gift to yourself and your partner. During the two weeks before you bleed—give or take a few days, depending upon the length of your cycle—hormones shift, energy intensifies or diminishes. Your estrogen peaks with ovulation and then declines. Your progesterone rises after ovulation and falls with your flow of blood. Your libido ebbs and flows to your own unique rhythm. Making love during this time, when you may be more open, more vulnerable than at other times in your cycle, can promote healing and deepen the connection between you and your partner.

The female orgasm, uncensored, especially by the mental constructs we create to translate expectations, demands that we open our body, our heart, and surrender to the one with whom we share the experience. And if initially we cannot get our mind out of the way, deep orgasm catalyzes this for us and everything else dissolves. This act of surrender opens a gateway to a deeper understanding of oneself and facilitates the opportunity, if we choose to seize it, to transcend the stress of our everyday lives and step into being fully present with another, even if the other is yourself alone.

Oriental medical tradition suggests that making love with penile penetration, and being orgasmic during the actual time a woman bleeds, is contraindicated. This is not because it is messy or dirty, or that it is bad for menstrual blood to come in contact with another human being. The belief stems from the physiologically energetic action that occurs in women during orgasm. The action of shedding the endometrial lining of our uterus travels downward and out of the body; the energy of orgasm for women draws upward, even in the presence of the flow of amrita, the female ejaculation. These two actions appear to conflict with each other.

Menstrual blood has historically carried connotations of mystery, contamination, magic, fear of the unknown, curses, fear of disease, tragedy or elation because of the lack of conception, the risk of death if out camping in the wild or swimming in the ocean, potential fertility signified by youth, and being unclean. In many native cultures, a menstruating woman is forbidden to participate in certain ceremonies, while in other cultures a woman in her bleeding moon is revered because of the power she wields while she bleeds. Some women actually use their blood during a ceremony, or as a nutrient to nourish the plants in their gardens.

Also bear in mind that if a woman carries a sexually transmitted disease—an STD such as hepatitis C, herpes simplex, or HIV, the AIDS virus—she potentially infects through intercourse, and the risk for this increases during her menses. (*Note:* It is important that you *not* have unprotected sex if you are not in an exclusive, mutually monogamous relationship, or if you know you or your partner carries an STD.)

Beyond mythologies, beyond beliefs, trust your intuition to direct you as to when it's okay for you to make love and when it does not serve you to do so. Let the energy of your physical, emotional, mental, and spiritual bodies assist you with your inner knowing, your natural rhythms, which ebb and flow as normally as do your hormones. Embrace another opportunity, in this dance we call life, to know thyself.

STRESS REDUCTION AND TIME OUT

Women in our modern world consistently sustain a high-stress threshold—maintaining homes, caring for and raising children, sustaining professional lives and jobs both inside and out of the home. One definition of stress in *Merriam-Webster's Collegiate Dictionary* (tenth edition) is *a physical, chemical, or emotional factor that causes bodily or mental tension and may be a factor in disease causation*. As women, we tend to internalize much of the strains and tensions we encounter in daily life in order to cope with the tasks we need to accomplish each day.

Worrying about what may or may not happen is one of the ways we create more stress for ourselves. Focusing on anything other than this moment and what this moment requires causes you to lose the present and possibly spin off into a scenario of a potentially fictitious future. Center on what appears to be real, right now, and do not worry about the future—you can deal with that when you get there. Write down what your distraction seems to be about and why it grips your attention. If you discover some underlying fear, confront it and try to discern if the fear has a connection to your current base reality.

Notice what upsetting things you tend to focus on that induce a physically and/or emotionally stressful response. Do you worry over possible future events, or do you fret over what has been? When we beat ourselves up over how we have handled an event or any scenario, we relive it. This holds little value, especially if you are in a PMS state of mind, other than to clarify other possibilities for some other unknown time, which may or may not occur. Yes, we can choose to learn from a situation. But the learning does not include playing it over and over again in our minds until we feel sick to death with what happened. It is no longer your reality, because it has passed. Know that in any given situation you have the opportunity to bring your best, authentic self to it. Is it possible that you could have handled things differently? Perhaps. But if you, in that moment, could have really handled things differently, don't you think you would have?

Don't worry over something that's going to happen in the future. Things are seldom how we imagine them. The very act of worrying demands that you concentrate on the object or concern. By the laws of nature, movement follows energy, energy follows attention. Do you really want to hold your attention on the antithesis of what you desire, the worry? Let go when appropriate or take action when it is needed.

Freeing your mind of false or unrealistic expectations or limitations, and choosing to be present with what is, reduces stress tremendously. Changing how you perceive your reality by shifting your attention to what is working in your life, rather than what is not, instantly evokes positive thoughts. Find the balance between when to take action and when to simply let something go.

If you live with other people, do you find time to be alone? Do you spend your alone time in bed trying to escape stress through sleep? Do you come home to an empty house after a stressful day at work and collapse and escape into a book, a bottle, or TV? We all need time to decompress, time when nothing is required of us by anyone.

You need to find time alone, time just for you, to be with yourself and to do whatever you want to do to nourish your being, because this is essential to your physical, mental, and spiritual health. Some things are only revealed within the confines of solitude. Make a list of the things you can do for yourself that inspire you and make you feel good about yourself. Have you been telling yourself that one of these days you are going to start a journal, begin a meditation practice, pick up painting watercolors, take a dance class, or make use of the exercise equipment in the nearby gym or community center? Now is the time to do it. Find time to spend with yourself and discover the mysteries within without trying to solve or fix them. Approach yourself with the compassion you would bring to a dear friend. Listen without judgment to the woman who dwells within you and who longs to be heard.

For the woman who finds it quite the challenge to make time for herself, try specific relaxation techniques. Consider a massage once a week, and rather than chatting away with your masseuse, relax under the therapeutic touch and just receive nurturing from another.

ACUPUNCTURE

Acupuncture, because of the use of needles, may not sound relaxing or therapeutic to those of you unfamiliar with the experience. But not only does acupuncture have a therapeutic value in the treatment of PMS, it also relaxes you, if you'll allow it to, and the very tiny needles, in the skilled hands of your acupuncturist, do not cause pain. Many PMS symptoms, if they do not require actual hormonal supplementation, can be resolved with acupuncture.

AROMATHERAPY

Essential oils containing phytohormones, inhaled and dabbed onto your skin, soothe some PMS symptoms, but aromatherapy, soothing scents breathed in while taking a hot bath by candlelight, works its magic anytime. Don't forget to actually take the time to do this simple, effective relaxation while you are distracted by PMS. I could give you a list of all the lovely scents available, but going to a shop—they're also found in most whole-food stores—and finding the ones you love is much more fun. You can also explore information provided at websites, although it lacks the olfactory sensory input. Try *www.frontiercoop.com/*.

If your nose appreciates the scent, trust it. Young Living has some interesting combinations of essential oils designed to address specific needs and concerns, and can be found at *www.youngliving.com*.

Here are some examples of essential oils naturally containing phytohormones that assist through the sense of smell.

- *Bergamot, Citrus bergamia,* has an aroma that is fresh, lively, fruity, and sweet; a lovely deodorizer, it produces the aromatherapy benefits of uplifting, inspiring, and helping to build self-confidence.
- *Cedarwood, Cedrus atlantica*, gives off a woody, oily scent and is sometimes described as slightly animal-like, with the aromatherapy values of stabilizing, centering, and strengthening the mind and mood.
- *Cinnamon Bark, Cinnamomum zeylanicum,* permeates with a warm, spicy effect, and gives the aromatherapy benefits of comforting and warming.
- *Clary Sage, Salvia sclarea,* generates a spicy, bittersweet aroma with the aromatherapy benefits of centering, euphoria, and enhancing visualization.
- *Sweet Fennel, Foeniculum vulgare var. dulce,* emits a sweet, earthy, aniselike aroma, and offers the aromatherapy qualities of nurturing, supporting, and restoring.
- *Geranium, Pelargonium graveolens,* releases a powerful, roselike fragrance with fruity, minty undertones, and the aromatherapy benefits of soothing, lifting moods, and balancing.
- *Ginger, Zingiber officinale,* has a warm, spicy, woody odor, with the aromatherapy effects of warming, strengthening, and anchoring.

- *Jasmine, Jasminum grandiflorum,* emits a full, rich, honeylike sweetness, sensual and romantic, with the aromatherapy benefits of calming and relaxing.
- *Lavender, Lavandula angustifolia,* exudes a sweet, balsamic, floral scent with the aromatherapy benefits of balancing, soothing, normalizing, calming, relaxing, and healing.
- *Neroli, Citrus aurantium,* has a very strong, refreshing, spicy, floral aroma with the aromatherapy benefits of calming and soothing, as well as its sensual qualities.
- *Sandalwood, Santalum album,* has a sweet, woody, warm, balsamic aroma with the aromatherapy benefits of relaxing and centering, and it has sensual qualities.

EXERCISE

The act of creating movement in your body—exercise—is another way to shift your perception of life and immediately transform the moment and your energy. Exercise releases endorphins, peptides secreted in your brain that have a pain-relieving effect similar to that of morphine; especially during PMS, they offer release or at least a reprieve. Be kind to yourself if you have not consistently exercised for some time, and be realistic with what you choose as your new exercise pattern. Pumping hard, especially when you're out of practice, can cause more harm than good and discourage you from trying something that might serve you better. Just before your period is not the time to take on a new heavy-duty workout program. As with anything else, you must find your own rhythm.

Make a realistic commitment to yourself to begin moving your body on a regular basis. Yoga is an ideal choice; it not only offers stretching, but there are postures that actually relieve some PMS symptoms. There are many different kinds of yoga. If you have never practiced it before, find a beginner class with a competent, compassionate instructor with whom you connect.

Explore whatever form of exercise attracts you. Hate to exercise? Walk. Step out your door and take a walk. And while your feet make contact with the earth, even if it's concrete, breathe in and pay attention to everything within your visual field. Hear the pleasant sounds as well as those that disturb. A walking meditation serves to center and calm your mind and stimulate your body.

Try putting on some good music at home and dance however the music moves you. No one is watching. Get together with a friend who also wants to exercise and rent several exercise videos. Find the ones you like. Make it fun. Because if you do not find a way to enjoy it, you are likely not to bother no matter how much you tell yourself you need it. These suggestions may help mitigate symptoms, but remember, if your symptoms are severe, and due to inadequate production of progesterone, you need a hormonal adjustment.

RX SUMMARY FOR PMS

1. Compounded phytogenic natural progesterone therapy, taken twice a day:

   - Dosage based on your hormonal analysis, which may include other hormones, or
   - For moderate to severe PMS, 100 mg of progesterone on days 12 or 14 to 28
   - For milder PMS, 50 mg of progesterone on days 14 to 28

In addition to phytogenic hormone therapy, you may want to consider augmentation with:

2. Diet high in protein and fiber and low in carbohydrates, sugar, and caffeine
3. Homeopathic remedies; dosages usually range between 30C and 200C, two to four times daily, as needed.

   - Apis
   - Belladonna
   - Chamomilla
   - Nux Vomica
   - Pulsatilla

- Sepia, or
- Your constitutional remedy

4. Herbal formulas

- Chinese herbals
    Bupleurum and Tang Kuei Formula
    Free and Easy Wanderer Plus
    Tang Kuei and Peony Formula
    Beauty Pearl
    Dong Quai/Tang Kuei
- Western herbals
    Black Cohosh
    Chasteberry
    Cramp Bark
    Damiana
    Dandelion Root
    Evening Primrose Oil
    Feverfew
    Gingerroot
    Licorice Root
    Oregon Grape Root
    Sarsaparilla Root
    Wild Yam Root

5. Vitamins and minerals—find a good formula that includes

- B complex
- Calcium (1,200 mg)
- Magnesium (600 mg)
- Folic acid (800 mcg)
- Vitamin A (10,000 IU)
- Vitamin C (750–1,000 mg)
- Vitamin D (400 IU)
- Vitamin E (800 IU)
- Selenium (150 mcg)

- Zinc (45 mg)
- Essential fatty acids (EFAs)

6. Orgasms
7. Stress reduction, massage
8. Make time for yourself, alone.
9. Acupuncture
10. Aromatherapy with phytohormones

- Bergamot
- Cedarwood
- Cinnamon Bark
- Clary Sage
- Fennel, sweet
- Geranium
- Ginger
- Jasmine
- Lavender
- Neroli
- Sandalwood

11. Exercise—yoga, dance, swim, tai chi, walk

The checklist on page 76 gives you the opportunity to look at some obvious disturbances common to millions of women. If you find yourself nodding yes to some of these complaints, you may want to photocopy the checklist, fill it out, and take it to your next appointment with the practitioner with whom you are working, specifically on your GYN-related health concerns.

WOMAN'S HEALTH APPRAISAL

NAME / AGE / DATE:

CHECK ANY THAT YOU EXPERIENCE 1–2 WEEKS BEFORE YOU BLEED:

- ☐ Anxiety
- ☐ Irritability
- ☐ Nervous tension
- ☐ Breast pain/tenderness
- ☐ Breast swelling
- ☐ Abdominal bloating
- ☐ Feeling shaky
- ☐ Heart palpitations

- ☐ Weight gain
- ☐ Water retention
- ☐ Increased appetite
- ☐ Depression
- ☐ Craving sweets
- ☐ Fatigue
- ☐ Insomnia
- ☐ Mood swings

- ☐ Headaches
- ☐ Forgetfulness
- ☐ Feeling withdrawn
- ☐ Acne
- ☐ Feeling self-destructive
- ☐ Feeling aggressive
- ☐ Sleep disturbances
- ☐ Night sweats

CHECK ANYTHING THAT OCCURS WHILE YOU ARE BLEEDING:

- ☐ Cramping
- ☐ Sharp pain
- ☐ Dull aching
- ☐ Diarrhea
- ☐ Headaches
- ☐ Weight gain

- ☐ Nausea, vomiting
- ☐ Low backache
- ☐ Upset stomach
- ☐ Mood swings
- ☐ Depression
- ☐ Accident prone

- ☐ Difficulty concentrating
- ☐ Painful/swollen breasts
- ☐ Decreased productivity
- ☐ Unusual fatigue
- ☐ Irritability
- ☐ Painful intercourse

CHECK ANY THAT DESCRIBES YOUR CYCLE:

- ☐ Heavy prolonged bleeding, on time
- ☐ Bleeding lasting longer than 5 days
- ☐ Frequently skipped periods
- ☐ More than 36 days between cycles
- ☐ Unusually light flow
- ☐ Vaginal dryness, itching, burning

- ☐ Irregular periods
- ☐ Frequent periods
- ☐ Frequent urination
- ☐ Bleeding between periods
- ☐ Absence of period for 3 months or more
- ☐ Vaginal discharge

CHECK ANY THAT YOU EXPERIENCE ANYTIME THROUGHOUT THE MONTH:

- ☐ Dizziness
- ☐ Irritability
- ☐ Anxiety
- ☐ Headaches
- ☐ Bone pain
- ☐ Dry skin
- ☐ Shakes
- ☐ Decline in vital energy and sense of well-being

- ☐ Chronic fatigue
- ☐ Memory problems
- ☐ Hot flashes
- ☐ Mood swings
- ☐ Night sweats
- ☐ Abnormal sweating
- ☐ Food problems

- ☐ Change in sexual desire
- ☐ Difficulty with orgasm
- ☐ Painful intercourse
- ☐ Loss of muscle tone
- ☐ Joint/muscle pain
- ☐ Trouble concentrating
- ☐ Digestive disturbances

- ☐ Chills
- ☐ Anger
- ☐ Depression
- ☐ Insomnia
- ☐ Pelvic pain
- ☐ Urinary pain
- ☐ Flatulence

OTHER CONCERNS:

HORMONE PING-PONG

PROGESTERONE DEFICIENCIES

PREGNANCY AND MISCARRIAGE

Phoebe's story, age thirty-eight

"I really still want to get pregnant, have a family," Phoebe cried when she came to see me for the first time. At thirty-eight years old, she had miscarried in her first trimester. She had what is technically termed a spontaneous abortion, a common event that happens for no apparent reason, her doctor told her. When I suggested we evaluate her hormones, she hesitated.

> I have very regular periods. I never experience PMS. What could be wrong with my hormones?

Not all hormone imbalances affect the regularity of the cycle. Sometimes the symptoms are quite subtle. She humored me and decided on a serum analysis because her insurance covered it. According to her blood levels, her progesterone was in the low range of normal. We also checked for other possible causes that might have prevented her from remaining pregnant. These tests were all normal.

The first prescription I put her on is what I consider a standard dosage of progesterone, 100 mg twice a day for twenty-one days of the month. Six months went by before I saw her again.

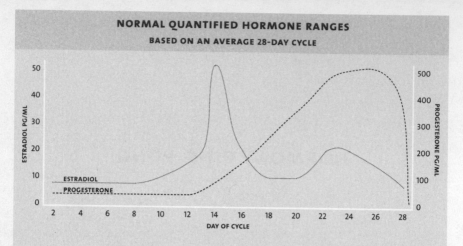

NORMAL QUANTIFIED HORMONE RANGES
BASED ON AN AVERAGE 28-DAY CYCLE

PREMENOPAUSE:	FOLLICULAR DAYS 1–13	PREOVULATORY DAYS 14–15	OVULATION DAY ~14	LUTEAL DAYS 16–CYCLE ENDS
Estradiol:	5–13 pg/ml	10–30 pg/ml	45–145 pg/ml	7–20 pg/ml
Progesterone:	20–100 pg/ml	20–100 pg/ml	20–100 pg/ml	65–500 pg/ml

NON CYCLE DEPENDENT HORMONES

Estriol:	< 3 pg/ml
Estrone:	Not established for below 40 years old
DHEA and DHEAS:	3–10 ng/ml
Testosterone:	8–20 pg/ml = Normal
	< 5 pg/ml = Depressed
	5–7 pg/ml = Borderline Low
	> 21 pg/ml = Elevated

POSTMENOPAUSE (NO CYCLE):	NO NHRT/HRT	PHYSIOLOGIC TARGET RANGE
Estradiol:	1–4 pg/ml	5–13 pg/ml
Estriol:	7–18 pg/ml	14–38 pg/ml
Estrone:		38–68 pg/ml (40–49 yrs)
		26–64 pg/ml (50–59 yrs)
		35–65 pg/ml (> 60 yrs)
Progesterone:	5–95 pg/ml	100–300 pg/ml
DHEA:	3 = Borderline Low	3–10 ng/ml = Normal range
	< 3 = Depressed	
Testosterone:		8–20 pg/ml

I stopped taking the progesterone. I didn't feel any difference and it sort of scared me to think about taking a hormone, even a natural one. Actually, I only took it for about nine days. But I also haven't gotten pregnant.

The blood test suggested a progesterone deficiency, but it was not specific enough. When a woman's blood is tested on a serum level, it measures the level of the hormone circulating in her bloodstream at the time the blood is drawn. A woman's hormones fluctuate throughout her cycle. But stress, traveling, altitude changes, inhaling the scent of someone who turns us on sexually, a change in a relationship or a new relationship, diet, weight loss or gain, and many health conditions influence our hormones and may alter the balance even within a single day.

Phoebe agreed to do the monthlong salivary analysis. This showed what Phoebe's progesterone levels were doing throughout her entire cycle—dropping too low too soon and bottoming out altogether before she bled. Often this can cause radical PMS, though not in Phoebe's experience.

Phoebe's progesterone fell short and too early in her cycle. In addition, her estrogen peaked too early. Although she hesitated when I first suggested a regime of natural progesterone, she decided to try this approach before considering fertility drugs. After one month of taking 25 mg of progesterone beginning on day two of her cycle through day fourteen, then increasing to 50 mg, to 100 mg, and then decreasing to 75 mg, Phoebe arrived rather nervous one day.

"My period's two days late, and I think I'm pregnant." The test agreed, and we wanted her to stay that way for forty weeks. Around the third month, Phoebe seemed distracted, almost sad.

I'm really scared. I'm afraid to feel happy about being pregnant, afraid of being attached to this baby. What if I lose this baby, too? What if something goes wrong?

There are never guarantees in any pregnancy. However, monitoring Phoebe's progesterone levels throughout her pregnancy offered a specific guideline for the dosage she needed in order to carry this baby. Whenever I tried to taper off the progesterone, she would develop cramping and low back pains, or headaches. Keep in mind, when extracted from wild yam into a powder, dissolved in olive oil, and encapsulated, this progesterone is identical to the progesterone we make in our own bodies. This made it safe for Phoebe and her baby, too.

She continued to take progesterone until the day before she gave birth to a very normal, healthy baby girl, thirty-seven and a half weeks after initiating natural progesterone therapy. When she came in to show me her baby and to reevaluate her hormonal balance, she looked radiantly beautiful.

If you have been trying to become pregnant and you either have been unable to conceive or have miscarried for no known reason, do an extensive hormonal panel that includes each hormone and consider a thyroid and adrenal panel as well. Progesterone deficiency can be a result of another dominant hormone such as testosterone overriding and suppressing your normal progesterone production.

RX SUMMARY TO SUPPORT PREGNANCY

1. Evaluate your hormones by salivary or twenty-four-hour urine analysis.
2. Compounded phytogenic natural progesterone therapy, taken twice a day:

   - Dosage based on your hormonal analysis, or
   - Progesterone: 25–35 mg on days 2 to 14; 50 mg on days 15 to 21; 100 mg on days 22 to 24; 75 mg on days 25 and 26; 50 mg on days 27 and 28, until pregnant
   - Reevaluate progesterone levels throughout pregnancy and adjust the dosage as needed.

In addition to phytogenic progesterone therapy, you may want to consider augmentation as follows:

3. Good nutrition is essential. If you're trying to conceive, treat yourself as though you're already pregnant and eat a diet high in protein and fiber and low in carbohydrates and sugar.
4. Chart your cycle (*see* Fertility Awareness Cycle graph, page 84).

5. Homeopathic remedies to support pregnancy and prevent miscarriage, including:

- Your constitutional remedy
- Apis
- Belladonna
- Caulophyllum
- Helonias
- Ipecacuanha
- Kali Carbonicum
- Plumbum
- Sabina
- Sepia
- Thlapsi
- Ustilago
- Viburnum

6. Herbal support

- Fenugreek to promote fertility
- Hollyhock to prevent miscarriage
- Red Raspberry Leaf to support pregnancy

7. Vitamins, minerals, and antioxidants in a good prenatal formula that does not induce nausea is essential and should include:

- Calcium (1,000–1,200 mg)
- Folic acid (1 mg)
- Beta-carotene (4,000 IU)
- Magnesium (500–600 mg)
- Vitamin A (4,000 IU)
- Vitamin B-1 (3.4 mg)
- Vitamin B-2 (3.4 mg)
- Vitamin B-12 (12 mcg)
- Vitamin B-5 (20 mg)
- Vitamin B-6 (10 mg), with a separate 50 mg of B-6 taken twice a day with morning sickness (but not on an empty stomach)
- Niacinamide (40 mg)

- Biotin (300 mcg)
- Vitamin C (500 mg)
- Vitamin D-3 (400 IU)
- Vitamin E (400 IU)
- Vitamin K (65 mcg)
- Iron (60 mg)
- Copper (2 mg)
- Iodine (175 mcg)
- Manganese (1.2 mg)
- Selenium (12.5 mcg)
- Molybdenum (25 mcg)
- Chromium (25 mcg)
- Inositol (50 mg)
- Quercetin (6 mg)
- Phosphorus (100 mg)
- Zinc (25 mg)
- Essential fatty acids (EFAs)

Note: Higher doses are needed with specific deficiencies or other conditions, as in anemia.

8. Orgasmic expressions
9. Stress reduction, relaxation, massage
10. Make time for yourself, alone.
11. Acupuncture
12. Aromatherapy
13. Exercise—yoga, tai chi, dance, swim, walk

The Fertility Awareness Cycle graph on page 84 is best used with a basal thermometer. You can photocopy that page and make several copies to work with each month. Basal temperatures reflect the body in resting conditions and measure lower than other times during the day. Consider the first day of your menstrual flow as Day 1.

This method can help you determine when you ovulate. Once the ovum has been released during ovulation, the basal temperature will be 0.4°–0.6°F higher during the second half of your cycle than in the first half. During ovulation, your basal temperature will show a sharp rise to a peak, followed by an immediate drop.

INSTRUCTIONS

1. Purchase a special basal body thermometer, as it is easier to read incremental changes.
2. Before you go to sleep, shake down the thermometer and place it on your bedside table so that you can reach it first thing upon awakening with the least amount of effort or movement.
3. When you awaken, before you even get out of bed, place the thermometer under your tongue with your mouth closed, for five clocked minutes.
4. Record the reading by placing a dot on the graph under the appropriate day of your cycle and note the date. Connect the dot to the previous day's dot by drawing a straight line.
5. Day 1 of your cycle equals the first day of actual menstrual blood flow. Begin a new graph with *each* day 1.
6. Circle each dot on the days you make love.
7. If you have a restless night, become ill, catch a cold, or awaken an hour earlier or later than usual, make a notation to that effect, as these will affect your temperature reading.
8. Charting your cycle for two or three months will help show your ovulation pattern.
9. Temperature fluctuations can occur due to illness or specific activities. Consult your physician or practitioner for further clarification.

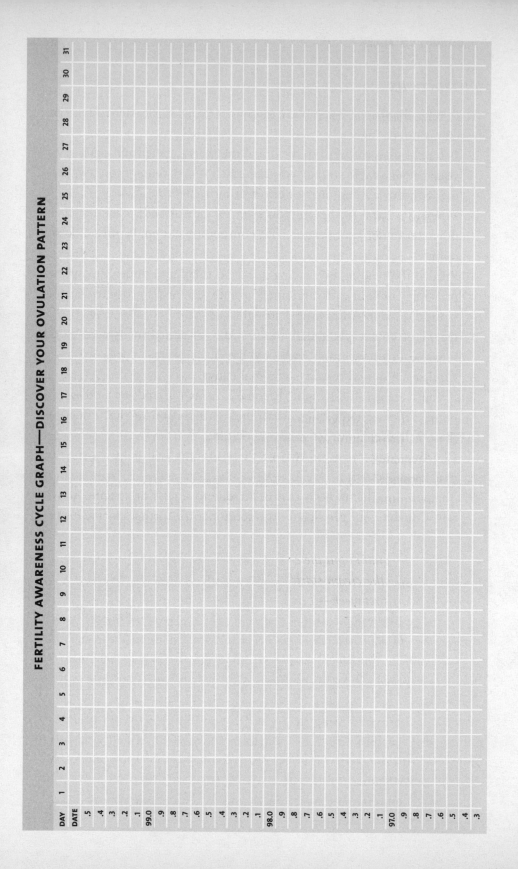

FERTILITY AWARENESS CYCLE GRAPH—DISCOVER YOUR OVULATION PATTERN

DAY	1	2	3	4	5	6	7	8	9	10	11	12	13	14	15	16	17	18	19	20	21	22	23	24	25	26	27	28	29	30	31
DATE																															
.5																															
.4																															
.3																															
.2																															
.1																															
99.0																															
.9																															
.8																															
.7																															
.6																															
.5																															
.4																															
.3																															
.2																															
.1																															
98.0																															
.9																															
.8																															
.7																															
.6																															
.5																															
.4																															
.3																															
.2																															
.1																															
97.0																															
.9																															
.8																															
.7																															
.6																															
.5																															
.4																															
.3																															

ABSENT CYCLES

Adrienne's experience, age thirty-two

> *I'm only thirty-two years old and I haven't had a period in three months. What does this mean? I thought maybe I was pregnant, but the urine test said no. My breasts are so swollen, I look like I could be nursing. And my breasts hurt so much, my boyfriend can't touch me without getting a scream instead of sweetness. Actually, I've been anything but sweet. It's like I've had PMS every day for the past two months.*

Adrienne had previously experienced an ectopic pregnancy. Concerned about this possibility, she held little trust in a home pregnancy test. We ran a quantitative beta HCG—the highly sensitive serum test that measures the amount of human chorionic gonadotropin (HCG) hormone in numerical value—just to be sure. As she suspected, Adrienne was not pregnant. She was experiencing amenorrhea, the absence of her menses. Insufficient production of progesterone caused her monthly cycles to cease. Fortunately, her remedy is an easy one. Ten percent progesterone cream, applied every twelve hours, reestablished her regular rhythm within two months. Within one month, her breast swelling and pain disappeared.

> *At first, I couldn't put the cream on my breasts because they were so sore. Once the cream started working—and I could notice a difference in the first week—it felt soothing to massage my breasts with it. Actually, Tim volunteered for that job. He was so grateful to have me back again he would have smeared it everywhere. I'm glad I wasn't pregnant . . . maybe someday, but not now. And I'm so glad it was not early menopause, as one friend suggested.*

Adrienne continued using the progesterone cream for twenty-one days of her cycle each month for the next three years. For Adrienne, supplementing with progesterone stabilized the regularity of her cycle, eliminated her PMS, and enabled her to feel normal.

Not all amenorrhea is caused by insufficient progesterone, preg-

nancy, or menopause. Excess testosterone can also prevent menstruation, as is apparent in some women athletes. Women who exercise to an
extreme for their own hormonal constitution may experience amenorrhea because they have essentially pumped up their testosterone to abnormally high levels while building muscle mass. These high levels of
testosterone suppress the production of progesterone. This does not
mean you must give up exercising, although you may want to reassess
the extent and form of your exercise, along with your motivation. This
is one of the ways your body tells you there's an imbalance.

Another cause of amenorrhea is the condition called anorexia ner-
vosa, defined by *Taber's Medical Dictionary* as "loss of appetite for food
unexplainable by local disease. It is a symptom of mental illness."
Women with anorexia sustain a state of malnutrition and lose so much
of their body weight that they cannot afford to lose blood each month.
A condition called polycystic ovaries, usually identified on a thorough
pelvic exam, can also cause the cessation of monthly bleeding.

Sustained stress—experienced physically, mentally, emotionally, or
spiritually—can alter a woman's hormonal balance and delay cycles,
cause them to be skipped, or, conversely, cause her to bleed more often.
Stress, especially when it continues over an extended period, results in
an unhealthy, sometimes hyperalert state, or burnout, which further
compromises the function of any aspect of the endocrine system, including the adrenals, ovaries, pituitary, parathyroid, and thyroid.

If you know you are not pregnant or menopausal, have not menstru-
ated for three consecutive months, and have tried treating yourself with
natural progesterone twice a day for twenty-one days and off for seven
days, for three months consistently, consider reevaluation from a professional perspective. In addition to a complete physical examination and
blood analysis, the serum prolactin, a hormone produced by the anterior
lobe of the pituitary gland, should be evaluated. Elevated prolactin levels suggest a pituitary tumor, which can be confirmed through an MRI.

RX SUMMARY FOR ABSENT CYCLES

1. Compounded phytogenic natural progesterone therapy, taken twice
   a day:

- Dosage based on your hormonal analysis, or
- Progesterone: 100 mg for twenty-one days, then discontinue for seven days to allow your period to flow. Continue this until a normal pattern has reestablished or for three months. Then:
- Progesterone: 25–35 mg on days 2 to 10; 50 mg on days 11 to 16; 75 mg on days 17 to 20; 100 mg on days 21 to 26; 75 mg for 2 days, or until menses

    Note: Some women find that taking 100 mg of progesterone throughout the month serves to keep their optimal balance.

In addition to phytogenic progesterone therapy, you may want to consider augmentation with:

2. Balanced nutrition with a whole-foods diet
3. Homeopathic remedies

    - Caulophyllum
    - China Officinalis
    - Cyclamen
    - Graphites
    - Ignatia
    - Kali Carbonicum
    - Pulsatilla
    - Sepia
    - Silicea
    - Tuberculinum

4. Herbals

    - Dong Quai
    - Nettle Leaf
    - Pennyroyal Tea

5. Vitamins, minerals, and antioxidants
6. Stress reduction, relaxation
7. Time out for fun, or other things you long to do for yourself
8. Acupuncture

9. Aromatherapy
10. Balanced exercise—not too much, not too little

TO BED BECAUSE OF MY HEAD

Migraines, headaches, the relentless pounding before, during, or after
we bleed . . . Drugs knock us out, send us to bed in a dark room to lie
still, undisturbed, while the world continues on. Hardly a satisfying way
to spend those days, unless we retain an unusual definition of downtime.
Most of us have things we want to accomplish and we don't want to sacrifice precious time to a migraine. Yet if you have ever experienced one,
you understand that while in the Vise-Grip, choices feel quite limited.

Madge's experience, age forty-nine

Madge brought her calendar in for her visit with me. Previously, she did
not know when the migraines began or why. I suggested there might be
a pattern to them and she could discover this quite easily if, on the same
calendar or journal in which she noted her cycle, she also tracked when
her migraines occurred.

> Look, Saundra . . . See all these months where my migraines came
> just before my period started. Now, since I've been taking the
> progesterone—and I'm doing it like you told me, the moment I feel
> it starting—no migraine this month, none here either. I really didn't
> think this little capsule of yams could stop it. You know me. I'm such
> a skeptic.

To abate a hormonally induced migraine, take 100 mg of progesterone at the very first sign of the onset of symptoms and every four hours
after that until every hint of it is gone. In Madge's case, her sudden drop
in progesterone triggered a migraine. Taking this a step further, by giving her gradually increasing doses of progesterone throughout her cycle
to reestablish a normal hormonal pattern, we halted the threat of migraines altogether.

Many women experience hormonal migraines. As their stories are
consistently similar, I chose to share this one as a common example. The
symptoms arise just before the period begins, during the first few days of

bleeding, or coincide with the most intense phase of the PMS. Almost all hormonally based migraines are triggered by the sudden reduction of progesterone production just prior to the onset of monthly bleeding.

Progesterone needs to build up to an adequate level and then decrease to initiate bleeding, the shedding of the endometrial lining. Some women develop headaches or migraines the first or last day of their cycle. These, too, are caused by a hormonal imbalance. If you experience regular headaches or migraines, chart when they occur and keep track of your cycle. If you see a pattern connecting the migraines to your cycle, in any phase, evaluate your hormones.

During the menopausal process, not all hormonal headaches are caused by a progesterone deficiency. At this stage of the delicate hormonal balance, the headache or migraine may be caused by insufficient estrogen. Try the progesterone approach first. But if your headaches and migraines do not respond to the progesterone, follow the directions in the summary for the biestrogen treatment.

RX SUMMARY FOR HORMONAL HEADACHES AND MIGRAINES

1. Compounded phytogenic natural hormone therapy, taken twice a day:

- Dosage based on your hormonal analysis, or
- Progesterone: 25–35 mg on days 2 to 14; 50 mg on days 15 to 21; 100 mg on days 21 to 26; 75 mg until onset of menses

In addition:

- Progesterone: 100 mg orally at the very first sign of the beginning of a headache, then every four hours as needed. Or:
- Progesterone: 10 percent cream, a fingerful massaged directly into the headache's point of origin, then every two to four hours as needed

If your headache/migraine does not respond to progesterone:

- Biestrogen: 1.25 mg in sublingual drops, take 1–2 drops at the first sign of headache, and every four hours, as needed. Or:

- Biestrogen cream: 5 mg per gram, massage a fingerful of cream as directed above for progesterone cream

In addition to phytogenic hormone therapy, you may want to consider augmentation with:

2. Balanced nutrition

- Whole foods free of refined sugars, flour, and cereal
- Organic, free-range poultry and fresh fish
- Avoid sulfites—sulfites trigger migraines, and are found, for example, in nonorganic red wine; sulfites may also be sprayed on salad bars at restaurants that do not serve organic veggies.
- Avoid all processed foods containing additives, preservatives, exogenous hormones, and chemicals.
- Watch your caffeine intake and minimize it.
- Drink at least one to two liters of pure water a day.

3. Homeopathic remedies (There are many; here are some to try.)

- Aconite
- Arnica
- Aurum
- Belladonna
- Bryonia
- Calcarea Phosphorica
- Gelsemium
- Iris
- Kali Bichromicum
- Nux Vomica
- Sanguinaria

4. Herbal support

- Black Cohosh
- Feverfew
- Lady's Mantle

- Primrose
- Sage
- Skullcap
- St. John's Wort
- Vervain
- Willow Leaves

5. Balanced multivitamin and mineral formula, plus an antioxidant formula
6. Stress reduction
7. Acupuncture
8. Aromatherapy

- Chamomile
- Lavender
- Rosemary

9. Exercise—yoga, breath-work meditation

ALLERGIC TO YOUR OWN PROGESTERONE?

Negative reactions to phytogenic natural progesterone are rare but can seriously disturb the woman who experiences them. Usually a woman is not aware that she has had adverse responses to her own progesterone unless she experienced this in pregnancy. The symptoms can be physical, mental/emotional, or a combination of both.

Abigail's story, age fifty

Twenty-four hours after taking her second dosage of 100 mg of progesterone, Abigail phoned me in hysterics.

> This happened to me when I was pregnant and I forgot to tell you about it. I haven't slept and I feel crazy, I mean really crazy! Suddenly I can't function or focus on anything. It's like the most intense episode of PMS. This sense of craziness started a few hours after I took the first dose. I had forgotten that I felt like this in pregnancy.

So I took the second dose twelve hours later, not realizing that it was what was causing me to feel like this. I haven't taken any more because I must be able to work.

Abigail's progesterone levels measured below normal, but taking the natural phytogenic progesterone affected her quite the opposite of how I expected it to. It matched exactly the way she felt during the rise in her own progesterone, and it was impossible to live with. After I reassured her that we would work out another approach and find the appropriate dosage for her, she calmed down.

I suggested we change her progesterone from the oral capsule to the transdermal or sublingual approach to give her more control of her dosage, and that we start with the lowest possible dosage. She chose the cream and began with what I consider almost a homeopathic amount, a fingernail full.

Over the next several months she worked up to one-sixteenth of a teaspoon. The normal dosage is one-quarter to one-half teaspoon when using 10 percent progesterone. Abigail continued with this dosage for several years, until she became menopausal and needed to add a biestrogen and DHEA, each in separate capsules, to her regime. I started her at a very low dosage of 0.625 mg biestrogen in consideration of her hypersensitivity to progesterone. As her hot flashes increased, we tried to slightly increase her progesterone, but she immediately complained of feeling crazy again.

Unlike most women I have worked with, Abigail tolerated the estrogens and the 5 mg of DHEA far better than progesterone. While she remained on this low dosage of progesterone, she felt normal and maintained adequate protection for her womb, because her estrogen remained opposed by some progesterone. Unopposed estrogen—estrogen taken without progesterone—can cause endometrial cancer in a woman who still has her uterus.

Aleta's story, age sixty-one
Aleta's experience was completely physical, manifesting in the form of recurrent symptoms of a bladder infection. She did not remember anything unusual in her pregnancy. It took a while for me to figure out what she had reacted to, partly because I began working with her long

after she became postmenopausal. When Aleta first came to me at age sixty-one, she was taking 0.3 mg of Premarin every other day and had discontinued her Provera because she did not "feel normal" by her definition. Due to this unopposed estrogen approach, her previous physician monitored her uterus with annual pelvic ultrasounds.

After we discussed other natural options, she decided to try the phytogenic hormones in a transdermal cream form. While taking Premarin and Provera, she continued to experience hot flashes and the absence of her libido. Her first natural formula included DHEA and testosterone along with estrogen and progesterone. Within one month, Aleta developed bladder infection–like symptoms and vaginal yeast; these were treated with corn silk, and by consuming much more water than she normally drank, taking acidophilus, and using a naturopathic vaginal suppository called Y-stat. She also took a good look at her stress management and began to get regular massages.

It was not until this scenario repeated itself that I considered the possibility of her reacting to her hormonal formula. The hormonal analysis clearly showed she absorbed each hormone except her progesterone, which measured less than 21 pg/ml. The normal physiologic target range for women is between 100 and 300, and for the postmenopausal woman who does not take any HRT the range is between 5 and 95.

Because of this reading I thought her problem was due to inadequate progesterone absorption, so I increased it, lowered the estrogens, and discontinued the DHEA and testosterone. However, this did not remedy her situation. Instead, Aleta developed sore breasts, low backache, and urinary urgency. Determined to take only natural hormones, she hung in with our fine-tuning process until I discovered what worked for her. I separated her hormones into two different forms, 25 mg of progesterone and 0.625 mg of biestrogen in an oral and sublingual approach. She kept track of how she felt when she increased her dosage.

Now, six years later, she enjoys feeling well on her formula of 0.625 mg of biestrogen and 25 mg of progesterone in a combination cream, and a DHEA of 2.5 mg per drop, four drops twice a day. In Aleta's situation, there were extended times when it appeared that she was taking the most appropriate formula for her, but then something would change internally to offset her balance. Often it was stress-related, and her stress took a variety of forms at different times. It was apparent that she did not like how the Premarin and Provera made her feel. Usually a woman feels good on the natural progesterone, which is quite dissimilar from the synthetic progestins. Aleta, however, had developed a sensitivity to progesterone in any form, and although her system requires it for optimal balance, she can take it only in low doses.

RX SUMMARY FOR PROGESTERONE SENSITIVITY

1. Compounded phytogenic hormone therapy, taken twice a day:

   - The lowest dosage of progesterone, along with a balanced ratio of any other hormones you may need based on your hormonal analysis and symptoms, or
   - Progesterone: 25–35 mg twice a day; begin with the cream or sublingual drops so you can easily adjust your dosage
   - Plus biestrogen, DHEA, and testosterone as needed

In addition to phytogenic hormone therapy, you may want to consider augmentation with:

2. Balanced nutrition
3. Homeopathic and herbal remedies (refer to sections specific to your reactive symptoms)
4. Balanced multivitamin and mineral formula plus an antioxidant formula
5. Stress reduction
6. Regular massages
7. Acupuncture
8. Aromatherapy to soothe symptoms
9. Exercise—yoga, meditation

ESTROGEN: EXCESS/DOMINANCE OR DEFICIENCY

The estrogen effect is detailed in Chapter 6, which deals with the menopausal process. But a note here on estrogen is important for those who will not begin to think about menopause for many years yet. Age is certainly a factor catalyzing the decline of estrogen levels. But what about the phenomenon referred to as *estrogen dominance*? When more estrogen than progesterone is produced throughout the entire cycle, estrogen dominance seems apparent.

Estrogen dominance is not age dependent. As you will see in the section on DHEA deficiency, Daire, who was twenty-one at the time and far away from menopause, experienced estrogen dominance. Which comes first, deficiency or dominance? This is a difficult question to answer. Too much estrogen can feel worse than too little to one woman and may not be noticeable to another. If her estrogens suppress the progesterone levels to an extent that a woman experiences an intensification of PMS (see symptom lists on pages 47–49), she may feel a strong loss of self or actually feel crazy.

Too much estrogen, her own or from an exogenous source, can have an impact on a woman's sense of well-being to such an extent that she may feel suicidal. Other symptoms of estrogen excess, and deficiency, include excessive weight gain, discussed at length in Chapter 5, and the symptoms correlating with other hormonal deficiencies. A woman can also maintain levels of normal estrogen production, according to her hormonal analysis, and still develop a hormonal deficiency.

RX SUMMARY FOR ESTROGEN DOMINANCE

1. Evaluate your hormones through either the salivary or twenty-four-hour urine analysis.
2. Compounded phytogenic natural progesterone therapy, twice a day:

   - The dosage based on your hormonal analysis, or
   - Progesterone: 100 mg twice a day for twenty-one days once a normal pattern is established
   - Progesterone: 25–35 mg on days 2 to 14; 50 mg on days 15 to 19; 75 mg on days 20 to 21 and on day 28; 100 mg on days 22 to 25

In addition to phytogenic progesterone therapy, you may want to consider augmentation with:

3. Adequate rest
4. A salivary or twenty-four-hour urine analysis to rule out adrenal exhaustion and thyroid dysfunction
5. A healthy, whole-foods diet
6. Homeopathic, your constitutional remedy, or try:

   - Apis
   - Belladonna
   - Caulophyllum
   - Chamomilla
   - China Officinalis
   - Cyclamen
   - Graphites
   - Ignatia
   - Kali Carbonicum
   - Nux Vomica
   - Pulsatilla
   - Sepia
   - Silica
   - Tuberculinum

7. Herbal support

   - Black Cohosh
   - Chasteberry
   - Cramp Bark
   - Damiana
   - Dong Quai
   - Evening Primrose Oil
   - Feverfew
   - Gingerroot
   - Licorice Root
   - Nettle Leaf
   - Oregon Grape Root
   - Pennyroyal Tea
   - Sarsaparilla Root
   - Wild Yam Root

8. Balanced multivitamins, minerals, and antioxidants
9. Take time to nurture yourself.
10. Stress reduction
11. Acupuncture
12. Aromatherapy
13. Exercise—yoga, walk, swim, tai chi

RX SUMMARY FOR ESTROGEN DEFICIENCY

1. Evaluate your hormonal status.
2. Compounded phytogenic hormone therapy, taken twice a day

   • Formula based on your hormonal analysis or symptoms
   • Refer to the Rx Summary at the end of Chapter 6

In addition to phytogenic hormone therapy, you may want to consider augmentation with items 3–22 found in the Rx summary at the end of Chapter 6.

DHEA DEFICIENCY

Do you feel fatigued more often than not? Have you noticed that your general sense of well-being seems to have evaporated along with your energy to do things you know are good for you, like exercise? Do you feel ensnared in the loop of being too exhausted to muster up the energy to exercise, even though you have heard that exercising will give you more energy? If so, you could be suffering from an inadequate amount of DHEA.

Hormones fluctuate based on many internal and external factors. And just as with any other hormone, depressed or deficient DHEA levels can deeply affect your life and your ability to function at your best. Before salivary and twenty-four-hour urine hormonal analysis became available, serum DHEA levels needed to be sent to special laboratories; they were expensive and quite unreliable. Now we can measure circulating DHEA levels with more precision.

Previously, due to ineffective testing mechanisms, I would consider supplementing a woman with DHEA based on whether she had lost her vitality and sense of feeling right with herself. Now I prefer to base my decision to supplement on a combination of how she feels and her numerical hormonal value. I obtain a baseline numerical measurement to first use as a guide but then use it for comparative analysis after a period of treatment to reevaluate its effectiveness.

Daire, age twenty-one

Daire was twenty-one when she came to me complaining of amenorrhea and extreme fatigue—too much for someone her age. Prior to her appointment she had worked with endocrinologists and gynecologists looking for answers, but no apparent pathology presented itself. Her salivary hormone test revealed abnormally high estradiol throughout the entire month, which dropped, instead of peaking, at the expected time of ovulation. Her progesterone levels were abnormally low over the complete testing period, except for an unusual peak on day ten. And her DHEA measured low at 3 ng/ml, whereas the normal range is 3 to 10. Daire's test suggested not only deficiencies in both her DHEA and progesterone levels, but also what Dr. John Lee has defined as estrogen dominance.

Daire's prescription of progesterone, combined with 5 mg of DHEA, was gradually increased throughout the month. On days two through fourteen, she took 35 mg of progesterone twice a day, 50 mg on days fifteen to eighteen, 75 mg for days nineteen through twenty-four, 100 mg on days twenty-five to twenty-eight, and then back down to 75 mg on days twenty-nine and thirty. In the first month, she noticed she felt less fatigued, but reestablishing a normal cycle took several months.

In my experience, after working with many women whose DHEA levels tested in the low range of normal or as depressed values measuring below the average parameters, fatigue persists as the most recurrent indicator of DHEA deficiency. To date, I have not seen a DHEA deficiency without a significantly low level of progesterone.

RX SUMMARY FOR DHEA DEFICIENCY

1. Establish the numerical baseline of your DHEA levels.
2. Compounded phytogenic hormone therapy, taken twice a day:

- Formula based on hormonal analysis or symptoms
- Start with 5 mg, or less if you are sensitive, of DHEA per dose, increasing in 2.5–5 mg increments. If you get up to 50 mg dosages and do not feel improvement, reevaluate your DHEA levels and the diagnosis.

With midafternoon fatigue:

- DHEA: 5–10 mg with an extra dosage before your energy takes the midafternoon plummet

In addition to phytogenic hormone therapy, you may want to consider augmentation with:

3. Adequate rest
4. A salivary or twenty-four-hour urine analysis to rule out adrenal exhaustion and thyroid dysfunction
5. A healthy, whole-foods diet
6. Homeopathic remedies

   - Apo-Strum
   - Calc Carb
   - Kali Iodatum

7. Herbal support

   - Ginseng and Astragalus Formula
   - Ginseng Nourishing Formula

8. Balanced multivitamins, minerals, and antioxidants
9. Stress reduction
10. Take time to nurture yourself.
11. Acupuncture
12. Aromatherpy
13. Exercise—yoga, walk, swim, tai chi

DHEA CONVERSIONS

Presently, DHEA is a readily available nonprescription item easily obtained by anyone, which has its advantages and disadvantages. The key point I want to make is that I actually do not think it is healthy for everyone to simply dose themselves with DHEA, especially with some of the higher dosages available. DHEA can convert to other hormones, not just when we need them but spontaneously and without apparent cause. And it can occur even in brands manufactured by companies that claim that their methodology prevents DHEA conversion. I have witnessed this in blood tests and salivary analysis.

Let's say, for example, that a woman who naturally maintains sufficient testosterone levels takes DHEA because she has heard it is good for preventing cancer. Unfortunately, the DHEA converts to excess testosterone and she develops facial hair. When this occurs, the facial hair does not simply go away when she discontinues taking the DHEA supplement. I have seen it take many months, added expense, and electrolysis before the beard disappears. Now that testing requires that you collect a sample of either your saliva or urine in the comfort of your own home, I strongly urge you to get a baseline of your hormonal profile before augmenting, particularly with any hormone other than progesterone.

Darcy's experience, age thirty-eight

Taking birth control pills all these years cannot be my best option. Especially since I haven't had sex for years, so preventing pregnancy is not an issue. My periods are excruciating whenever they decide to show up, and I feel tired all the time. Somehow, at thirty-eight, I did not expect to need a daily nap just to get through the day. Fortunately, I work at home and I can schedule it in.

Darcy wanted to try taking something natural. At the time we began working together, effective DHEA testing was not yet available. Because her symptoms suggested a DHEA and progesterone deficiency, I started her on a formula of 100 mg of progesterone with 5 mg of DHEA in each dose. During the next six months she felt better and had more energy. However, Darcy developed facial hair. Deleting the DHEA from her formula slowed the increase in the hair growth but did not make it go away. She needed to go through a series of electrolysis treatments to resolve this. In Darcy's situation, although she was symptomatic of a DHEA deficiency, the DHEA converted to testosterone.

Seven years later, Darcy, now menopausal, takes a low dose combination formula of 1 mg of biestrogen and 75 mg of progesterone twice a day. The excess facial hair did not return, nor has she tried taking any more DHEA, even though her most recent salivary hormonal analysis measured her DHEA at 4, which is considered borderline low, with normal ranging between 3 and 10.

RX SUMMARY FOR DHEA CONVERSIONS

1. Test your hormones before initiating DHEA therapy.
2. If you are already taking DHEA and experience any symptom that suggests excess of another hormone, retest your hormones.
3. Discontinue the DHEA and adjust your compounded phytogenic hormones according to your profile of excess hormones and symptoms.

In addition to phytogenic hormone therapy, you may want to consider augmentation with:

4. Options to balance out the symptoms of excess hormones:

   • Homeopathy specific to your concern; refer to progesterone deficiencies and estrogen and testosterone dominance
   • Herbal helpers that soothe your specific reactive symptoms
   • Electrolysis, as needed for excessive facial hair
   • Acupuncture
   • Aromatherapy

5. Balanced nutrition; avoid foods that exacerbate your symptoms
6. Balanced vitamins, minerals, and antioxidants
7. Stress reduction
8. Consistent regular, but not excessive, exercise

TESTOSTERONE DOMINANCE

In Part One, you learned about each hormone and may have newly discovered that testosterone, normally considered the major male hormone, is also essential to a woman's hormonal balance. However, too much testosterone often causes unpleasant side effects, such as excessive hair growth (especially facial), absent cycles, infertility, and increased feelings of anger or hostility.

Tessa's experience, age forty-two

> I don't know what's wrong with me. I feel edgy all the time. I hardly sleep. And my poor husband, I snap his head off daily. I really don't know what I'm so angry about. Life has some stress in it, whose doesn't? But mostly my life is good. Am I going into menopause?

And Tessa certainly felt testy when I first met her. She seemed agitated while we spoke and wanted answers yesterday. Her physical examination did not reveal any pathological conditions and she brought her recently taken blood work, which was all normal, with her for me to see. Although her cycles were regular at every thirty-two days, it seemed too much of a stretch to expect her to do the monthlong saliva hormonal analysis. She agreed that not only did she not have the patience to collect her samples on specific days throughout the month, she felt that if she did not get relief soon, her marriage might be compromised.

When her single vial test results arrived, I was not surprised by her exceedingly elevated testosterone level of 98 pg/ml, her suppressed progesterone of less than 20 pg/ml, and her normal estrogens and DHEA. For this particular lab, a normal female testosterone level range is 8–20 pg/ml, and the progesterone span is 100–300 pg/ml. Her treatment began with 100 mg of progesterone in an oral capsule that she took twice a day, beginning on day four of her cycle, then she doubled her dose beginning on day twenty-two through day twenty-eight, and then back down to the original dosage.

> I can hardly believe how much better I feel. Larry said I haven't been snapping at him—unless he deserved it. No more feeling like I have

a nasty case of raging PMS every day. And blessed be, I can sleep again! You can see that I'm not as jumpy as I was when I saw you three months ago.

I wanted to reevaluate her testosterone level to make sure the numerical values reflected her experience. She did a single salivary sample for testosterone and progesterone. The testosterone had come down to 23 pg/ml, which indicates a significant improvement even though it remained slightly elevated. Because the salivary test for progesterone measured within the normal range, I decreased her dosage to 100 mg of progesterone twice a day on days four through thirty-one.

Tamara's experience, age twenty-eight

Tamara stopped having periods when she was twenty-eight. Previously, she had taken birth control pills in an attempt to bring on a normal cycle. However, when she discontinued them, her periods did not resume. Aside from the amenorrhea, her spirits seemed low. "I just want to be normal," she told me.

Tamara's testosterone measured 42 pg/ml, with normal levels of estrogens and DHEA, and she had a progesterone level of 30 pg/ml. Her prescription of 100 mg of progesterone twice a day for twenty-one days and then off for seven days began after inducing her period to begin by following a progesterone withdrawal remedy. To accomplish this, she took 100 mg of progesterone four to six times a day, a higher than normal dose, for up to one week only, then she stopped taking anything hormonally influencing and went about her life as usual until her menses came. Sometimes a woman begins to bleed while taking this higher dose. If this happens, she is to stop taking the progesterone at that time rather than continuing the full course of one week. Others may begin to bleed at the completion of this course, or not for several weeks. The response time depends upon how long cycles have been absent and sensitivity to progesterone.

What a relief! It felt like there had been this tremendous buildup without a release. At first I just spotted for two days. Then I did actually flow into what seemed like a normal period.

For the next six months, Tamara continued taking progesterone. She wanted to work toward not taking anything hormonal to see if she could maintain a normal rhythm on her own. But she also did not want to undo the benefit she experienced. We began with limiting the time she took her progesterone to the second half of her cycle. From day fourteen through twenty-six, Tamara took 100 mg of progesterone twice a day, then on days twenty-seven and twenty-eight she took 75 mg twice a day. After following this regime for three months, Tamara discontinued her progesterone altogether and experienced normal cycles for several months until her stress level increased. When she skipped her menses, she resumed her progesterone therapy.

ACNE, BEARDS—YIKES, CAN THIS BE?

There are hormonal zones—in the hairline, below the mouth, on the chest, back, and shoulders—where acne appears cyclically. Regardless of age, we can develop nasty zits, unrelated to diet, that are indicative of hormonal problems. Growing extra facial hair, sprouting hairs around the nipples, extensive arm hair, or pubic hair extending densely down the thighs—testosterone zones—as well as acne in the hairline and on the back, alarms any woman who wants to feel feminine. However, specific areas of our face and body relate to either an excess of testosterone or a progesterone imbalance. These conditions are easier to correct when you understand the cause.

Helene, age nineteen

Helene hated her hairiness. Unlike some of her close friends who thought of her as Ms. Au Naturel, she considered her excess hair an unsightly embarrassment and far from feminine, far from normal. She pointed out each specific area that, in her opinion, seemed unnatural.

> Look, see how thick my hair is on my thighs. It's as though my pubic hair just keeps on going. Usually I wax it all off, but I wanted you to see how bad it really is. And look at my chin, and my arms . . . Lately my face is breaking out, right up here almost into my scalp, about one week before my moon starts, whenever that is. Nobody I know has hair that grows like this, except guys. I feel like a freak.

At nineteen, Helene felt extremely conscious of her appearance and was intolerant of feeling she looked different. Curiously enough, her testosterone level was only slightly elevated, at 27 pg/ml, with normal ranging between 8 and 20. As with every woman under my care whose testosterone level is elevated, her progesterone level measured below normal. In some women it remains unclear which imbalance happens first, the increase in testosterone or the decrease in progesterone. But this combination seems to be the predominant scenario. For Helene, there were no known genetically influencing factors, and she had neither cystic ovaries nor abnormal prolactin levels. Her cycles came irregularly and she confessed to feeling discontent and edgy much of the time.

From her description of her cycles, the lack of ovulation—anovulatory cycles—suggested testosterone dominance. She agreed to chart her cycle and keep track of how she felt in relation to her cycle. During her first cycle on progesterone, she noticed certain changes.

Well, I'm not a grump all the time. And it seems like my friends haven't been calling me that since I started taking this medicine. My moon started on time—what a surprise. But my hair has not stopped growing.

Helene's progesterone therapy graduated throughout her cycle, beginning on day two through day fourteen with 25 mg, increasing to 50 mg through day nineteen, 75 mg on days twenty and twenty-one, 100 mg on days twenty-two through twenty-five, then back to 75 mg on days twenty-six and twenty-seven, and 50 mg on day twenty-eight. She took her progesterone in oral capsules twice a day. The intention behind this approach for Helene was to augment her progesterone and encourage a normal pattern.

Although her excess hair did not disappear in that first cycle, she did experience some positive benefits. Sometimes side effects secondary to prolonged hormonal imbalances take time to resolve, as they did for Helene. In reviewing her memory of menarche, the onset of her first menses, and her perception of her physical self, she described being hypercritical. Her cycles never established a regular pattern, and from menarche on she had tended toward excessive hair growth. She said she had difficulty with the thought of this process taking longer to resolve, but she would try to be patient, as she did not want to take anything that was not natural as a part of her treatment.

> *I'll wax my entire body, if that is what I must do for now. I may not want to pollute my body with chemicals, but I also don't want to look like a descendant of Bigfoot either. Even though I don't want to have a baby at this time in my life, at least now I feel like there may be the possibility at some time in the future, when the time is right for me. I didn't realize I had been afraid that all this hair and wacky cycles might mean I wouldn't be able to have children. I think I read in some magazine that this could happen.*

Over the next several months, Helene began to notice a gradual decline in the denseness with which her hair grew. She wanted an overnight miracle cure, which this clearly was not. But it was significant improvement. She continued taking the progesterone, which established regular cycles, and felt better about herself. As of our last visit, she still was not ready to begin a family, but her fears of possible infertility had dissipated with her consistently regular cycles. Her facial hair turned to mild peach fuzz, and other areas of hair-growth normalized.

If you continue to have an elevated testosterone level after balancing your hormones, please see your gynecologist for a pelvic exam and ultrasound to rule out ovarian cysts, and also to consider further evaluation of the pituitary gland.

RX SUMMARY FOR TESTOSTERONE DOMINANCE

1. Compounded phytogenic natural progesterone therapy, twice a day:

   - Dosage based on hormonal analysis, or
   - Progesterone: 100 mg twice a day for twenty-one days, once a normal pattern is established

   If amenorrhea is present:

   - Progesterone: 100 mg four to six times a day for one week, under your practitioner's guidance

With irregular cycles, take graduated dosages:

- Progesterone: 25–35 mg on days 2 to 14; 50 mg on days 15 to 19; 75 mg on days 20, 21, and 28; 100 mg on days 22 to 25

In addition to phytogenic progesterone therapy, you may want to consider augmentation with:

2. Balanced nutrition
3. Consider options to balance out the symptoms of excess:

- Homeopathy specific to your concern
     Apis
     Belladonna
     Caulophyllum
     Chamomilla
     China Officinalis
     Cyclamen
     Graphites
     Ignatia
     Kali Carbonicum
     Nux Vomica
     Pulsatilla
     Sepia
     Silicea
     Tuberculinum
- Herbal helpers that soothe symptoms
     Black Cohosh
     Chasteberry
     Cramp Bark
     Damiana
     Dong Quai
     Evening Primrose Oil
     Feverfew
     Gingerroot
     Licorice Root
     Nettle Leaf
     Oregon Grape Root

> Pennyroyal Tea
> Sarsaparilla Root
> Wild Yam Root

- • Electrolysis, as needed for excessive facial hair
- • Acupuncture
- • Aromatherapy

4. Balanced vitamins
5. Stress reduction
6. Meditation or at least a time-out
7. Consistent, not excessive, exercise—yoga, tai chi, swim, walk

TESTOSTERONE DEFICIENCY

The primary symptom of testosterone deficiency is the loss of one's interest in sex, or decreased libido. This can happen to a woman at any age, particularly as she approaches perimenopause and menopause, and especially if her life sustains a high stress threshold over an extended period. When loss of libido either directly correlates with relationship problems with one's partner or manifests as remaining in a dysfunctional relationship beyond endurance, a testosterone deficiency is unlikely; the source is then more emotionally rooted. Also, remember that our creative energy links to our sexual energy. So even if we are not in a sexual relationship, it is important to maintain a healthy libido if for no other reason than to channel it into our inspiration, our vision, and the practical application of our ingenuity.

Other manifestations of testosterone deficiencies include loss of muscle strength and tone, loss of physical stamina, loss of bone mass, loss of energy and the sense of well-being, and loss of one's ability to make decisions easily and stand up for one's truth. So far, I have yet to see a woman with a testosterone deficiency have all her other hormones completely balanced and within normal parameters for her age and where she is in her cycle. Usually, if she is not yet menopausal, her progesterone will register below the normal range. And if she is menopausal, her estrogen and progesterone will most likely quantify below optimum levels. In either situation, her DHEA may also be out of balance.

Taryn, age thirty-three

I know I'm here to see you for my annual, but can I talk to you about another problem I'm having? I live with this gem of a man. He is sweet to me, makes communication a priority, and he is intelligent with a spiritual focus. My problem is . . . I couldn't care less if we make love or not. It's not that I'm afraid of getting pregnant. We used to make love all the time and I love connecting with him. I don't know what's causing this. I'm young and have always loved sex. It seems unusual to me because we get along great, we are definitely compatible in bed, and life is generally good.

She also noticed that she was feeling less "fired up" about things in her life. Whereas previously she had been quick to debate anyone she disagreed with, lately she could not remember arguing any point at all. At first she thought this resulted from a spiritual maturity that perhaps she had evolved into. But when she lost all interest in sex, she suspected something was wrong.

When I asked Taryn about her cycles, she described normal twenty-seven-day cycles with little experience of PMS. Evaluating her hormones revealed, much to her relief, that Taryn was not approaching perimenopause, at the age of thirty-three, but was suffering from two primary hormonal deficiencies: not quite enough progesterone and a severe lack of testosterone. Slightly lower than average, her progesterone levels followed the expected rising curve, peaking, then dropping off just before her menses. Her estrogens and DHEA levels also appeared within normal range, but her testosterone was depressed at 5 pg/ml. Remember, normal testosterone measured in a salivary analysis ranges between 8 and 20.

The goal was not to get Taryn to fight with everyone, or to negate her spiritual process. We aimed toward restoring her balance. Taryn's prescription for the first month consisted of three approaches: an oral capsule of 50 mg of progesterone; testosterone dissolved in olive oil at 1 mg per drop; and testosterone cream dosed at 10 mg per gram. She took the drops under her tongue, increasing or decreasing the dosage based on her energy level. And she applied one-quarter of a gram of cream directly to her clitoral area twice a day, in the morning after her shower and in the evening around dinnertime, for one month. This application infuses the alcohol-free testosterone precisely where it is needed the most. It is best not to use the testosterone cream just before making love, as this may interfere in lovemaking with oral sex. Some men notice a change of smells or tastes in the woman and may be turned off by it.

Richard is really excited about our treatment. It seemed to start working within a few days. I didn't know if it was because I massaged my clit twice a day or if the testosterone just kicked in quickly, but I started attacking my sweetie. After months of living like a monk, or so he said, he's feeling pretty good these days.

Three months of taking the oral progesterone and the sublingual testosterone brought her libido and her energy back to normal. Her testosterone levels stabilized at 12 and her progesterone levels normalized. Taryn discovered that her muscle tone improved as well, although she had not realized it had slackened.

This subject will be discussed more in Chapter 6 (see page 160). Even though testosterone deficiencies are most common during perimenopause and menopause, I wanted to include a sample story here unrelated to menopause. I feel it is important to understand that any woman at any age can be lacking in testosterone. Other conditions, especially immunodeficiency disorders such as candidiasis, chronic fatigue syndrome, and AIDS, may be accompanied by testosterone deficiencies.

RX SUMMARY FOR TESTOSTERONE DEFICIENCY

1. Compounded phytogenic hormone therapy taken twice a day:

   - Progesterone, biestrogen, and DHEA based on your hormonal analysis or symptoms
   - Testosterone: 5 mg in an oral or sublingual approach when the libido remains unaffected

   Or, if your libido has disappeared:

   - Testosterone cream: 10 mg/gm, *alcohol free,* applied twice a day to the clitoral area for one month, and as needed afterward

In addition to phytogenic hormone therapy, you may want to consider augmentation with:

2. A healthy, whole-foods diet
3. Homeopathic remedies

   • Aurum
   • Causticum
   • Graphites
   • Natrum Muriaticum
   • Sepia
   • Silicea

4. Herbal support

   • Black Cohosh
   • Chasteberry
   • Damiana
   • Dong Quai
   • Evening Primrose Oil
   • Gingerroot
   • Licorice Root
   • Nettle Leaf
   • Oregon Grape Root
   • Sarsaparilla Root
   • Wild Yam Root

5. Balanced vitamins, minerals, and antioxidants
6. Work with your sexual energy, and consider other possible causes for loss of libido.
7. Pay attention to your stress levels/management.
8. Look to your creative self and nurture her.
9. Rule out thyroid dysfunction and adrenal exhaustion.
10. Acupuncture
11. Aromatherapy
12. Consistent exercise

5

ESTROGEN RESERVES

WEIGHT GAIN AND HORMONAL IMBALANCE

Is it true that I will gain weight, like I did on Premarin, if I take natural hormones? When I took Premarin, within the first month, I began to look like that pregnant mare whose estrogen I was taking.

Estrogen lives in fat cells. When our estrogen levels start to decrease, Mother Nature—kindly, well-intended—begins to hoard fat with the idea of trying to preserve what precious estrogen reserves she can. This process takes time to reverse, but it is not hopeless.

Once a woman, weaving through the threshold of perimenopause and menopause, begins gaining weight, she despairs over the radical change in her image. No longer fitting into her clothes, she often treads down the path that takes her further away from the vibrant self she had grown to know and accept. Exercise fades, as does her energy. The less she exercises, the fatter she gets. The fatter she gets, the less inspired she feels. Hopeless, she eats more comfort foods and only exacerbates the problem at hand.

Not only the physical body responds to this weight gain. Putting on weight is sometimes an effective, unconscious way to create distance between oneself and one's sexual partner. The excess weight creates a physical barrier between two bodies during intimacy. Yet often this physical barrier is the reflection of unspoken, unresolved issues within the dynamic of the relationship. If it is not the partner in a relationship that gets pushed away, then it is usually creativity that suffers. Sexual energy and creative energy are directly linked through the same channels.

Independent of making love with a partner, if one's sexual energy is blocked, the lack of juiciness seems to interfere with our ability to be creative. When I refer to creativity, I am not only addressing the artist within. I am also including the potential for creative thinking and the bringing of our creative, resourceful selves into any activity we do, whether it is cooking a meal or adding another perspective to a project.

If you are living on Häagen-Dazs ice cream, cookies, or any other of the myriad comfort foods, your weight gain may have nothing to do with your hormones. You may be caught in a mind loop that reinforces negative eating patterns with hopeless thinking.

Faith, age forty-five

> I can't lose weight no matter what I do. I diet and diet and diet. Actually, I think I've tried every weight-loss diet out there . . . and look at me. I'm a very large, actually an extra-large.

Faith sobbed as she recounted all the different diet plans she had been on. Now she ate what she wanted when she wanted to or could find the time. I asked her what she eats for breakfast. She stared blankly for a moment, and then told me she had a cup of coffee, maybe two. By one-thirty or two in the afternoon she would pause long enough to grab a sandwich or something from a local fast-food smorgasbord—though she confessed there were days when a pastry carried her through the day.

> When I get home from my usually hectic day, I might have some chips and salsa, because by then I'm starving. And so is everyone else in the house—the dogs, the cats, the kids, my husband. So I've gotta get dinner made, pronto. On a good day, I'll broil a piece of ahi, steam rice and a veggie, or make a salad. But some nights we just order a pizza.

Does this eating pattern sound at all familiar? Even if you're not currently a size extra-large, have you been too busy to eat and eat well? Do you tell yourself you aren't hungry when you know you're running on empty? There is a plethora of dietary guidelines available, and if you resonate to a particular nutritional philosophy, it is possible to use what works from that information to create a plan tailored to your own specific needs.

We have all heard for many years now that breakfast is *the* most important meal of the day. Actually, it is *one* of them. I stress "one" because in my experience with thousands of women, many of whom do battle with their bodies and the food they take in, each meal is important, especially if you want to lose weight, keep the excess weight off, and maintain a healthy body. Some of what it takes to effectively transform our physical selves is to change our eating habits. This requires us to stop ingesting foods that feed fat cells and plump them out further. For most of us, this also means that we have to think differently about food. The other component compels us to begin a practical regimen of consistently moving the body.

Faith was also experiencing irregular cycles and breaking into occasional night sweats, which kept her from adequate rest. In addition to making changes in her eating habits, including discovering a new morning regime that included protein with her coffee, she also started taking 100 mg of progesterone twice a day.

> *I feel a difference! Immediately I began sleeping through the night. Even though the thought of food first thing in the morning gagged me, I've been managing one of those protein drinks after my coffee, instead of a pastry, and I'm not eating late at night. I've actually lost five pounds and it feels like it might stay off this time.*

Let's focus on not only what we put into our mouths and swallow, but also what we devour with our minds.

Cora, age forty-two

Cora, a beautiful woman in her early forties, shared her relationship with food this way:

> *I hate food! All of it! Every time I eat anything, even something healthy, strong feelings come over me. Sometimes it's guilt, other times the fear that springs to the surface of my mind is a bit scary.*

But the real clincher grabs me when I feel spiteful. It's as though I go into a state of revenge against my own body . . . This has gotten much worse since my periods became a bit irregular and I've started gaining weight.

I tested her hormones and discovered that although Cora was just approaching her forty-second birthday, her estrogen levels resembled those of someone postmenopausal, and her progesterone had bottomed out to a low flat line. It's no wonder Cora felt rather bizarre, though without the typical menopausal symptoms of hot flashes and night sweats. One month after she had been taking 2.5 mg of biestrogen with 100 mg of progesterone, she noticed some positive changes.

I'm feeling more like myself again, not such morose thoughts. But these ten extra pounds I've put on must go. My clothes don't fit and I've got some great things that I love to wear that make me feel good about how I present myself to the world. All I'm really fitting into are things that qualify me as a bag lady!

Three months later, Cora arrived for her visit wearing a fitted skirt and flattering blouse. She had lost the ten pounds and continued to maintain her current weight. Cora admitted she still wanted to increase her muscle tone. But since she had lost the weight, she noticed a change in her attitude toward the exercise she needed for toning. Now she felt ready to tackle what previously had felt insurmountable.

As we get older, particularly as we enter any stage associated with the menopausal process, metabolism slows down for most women. Some women can eat whatever and whenever they want regardless of their age, weight, or hormonal shifting and get away with it. But this is not common. Most women as they approach menopause find gaining weight easy and losing it more challenging. A slower metabolism plus the process of our bodies' wanting to create fat cells in which to store estrogen add up to unwanted pounds, unless we choose to make changes.

Hormonal balance can be an essential ingredient along with becoming mindful of how we eat in order to maintain our optimum weight. The decline of a woman's estrogen is like an internal alarm clock set to activate her fat concentrations to rise, especially in certain areas such as the upper arms, abdomen, hips, buttocks, thighs, and knees. These areas become more soft tissue locations rather than muscle mass, perfect storehouses for estrogen to settle in. This can lead to disconcerting transformations in one's body image. When we balance our hormones, we send our body the message that we do not need to retain extra fat cells to store estrogen for those hormonally lean times ahead.

Want to know what eating habits really work? What will help eliminate unwanted pounds and keep them off? Eat small and frequent meals, about the size of your hand, every two to three hours and not later than four hours before bedtime. This will increase your metabolism by fueling your internal burner, increasing your ability to burn calories and turn them into energy. Food is the body's major source of energy when we eat what the body needs. How do we learn what we need? One way is to simplify our diet, eat only quality foods, and eliminate the junk, the comfort foods. These are mostly carbohydrates and sugars.

"What is left for me to eat?" Cora had asked.

Protein: Eating small frequent meals of primarily a good, healthy source of protein, with fresh vegetables and some fruit, can change your life. If you are vegetarian, choose protein sources low in carbohydrates. Not every meal needs to be complex or require major preparation.

For the wildly busy woman, whether she gets lost in her professional world or the demands of motherhood, her body needs fuel for energy. Skipping breakfast, slugging down coffee, racing through the day and eating something on the go does not cut it in the long run. Even if you've gotten away with this approach for the past twenty or thirty years, you are unlikely to now as you enter this significant life transition.

SOME DIETARY OPTIONS

Begin by finding a protein powder that is low in carbohydrates, low in sugar, has a taste that is pleasing, and that you can digest without any bloating or flatulent side effects. Many on the market today contain 20 to 40 grams of protein per serving. Personally, I prefer whey protein over soy because, as I understand, from a Chinese medical perspective, according to the many doctors of Oriental medicine with whom I have spoken, it is not as damp as the soy protein. If you have a constitution in which you tend to run cold or cooler than everyone else in a room, foods that are considered damp can exacerbate this tendency.

For breakfast, consider whether you have the time or the desire to sit and chew a meal. If the answer is no, regardless of your reasoning, this is a great time to have that protein drink. You can get quite creative with these drinks or you can keep them simple. Here are a few recipes that are delicious.

Try not to add sugar, honey, or other sweeteners. If you really have a sweet tooth, add a few drops of stevia, which is a naturally occurring plant source of sweetness that contains no calories and does not stress the pancreas. So even those of you who live with candidiasis or diabetes can use it. A good supplier for stevia can be found at *www.rainforestbio.com/amazonherb/*.

PROTEIN DRINK RECIPES

MANGO DELIGHT

> 1 scoop protein powder, or at least 20 grams
> 1 fresh mango, peeled and cut into chunks
> 1 cup orange juice

Blend in the blender until smooth and frothy.

CREMESICLE

> 1 scoop protein powder
> ½ cup orange juice
> 1 cup nonfat vanilla yogurt
> Pinch freshly grated nutmeg

Blend in the blender.

APPLE HAVEN

> 1 scoop protein powder
> ½ cup unsweetened applesauce
> 1 cup unsweetened apple juice
> ¼ teaspoon ground cinnamon

Blend in the blender.

TROPICAL ECSTASY

1 scoop protein powder

1 banana

½ papaya, peeled and cut into chunks

½ cup strawberries, hulled

Coco water (the clear liquid from inside a coconut)

½ cup chopped pineapple

Blend thoroughly, adding more coco water if needed.

For those of you who may be dealing with candidiasis, and cannot have even fruit sources of sugar or dairy, try any of the following, experimenting with variations as well. For more information on the best dietary approach to assist healing candidiasis, read *The Body Ecology Diet* by Donna Gates, or go to *www.bodyecologydiet.com/*.

ALMOND MILK

Soak almonds in filtered water either overnight or for eight hours. Remove the skins. If the skins remain tight even after the soaking, boil the almonds in enough water to cover, allow to cool, and then peel them. In a blender, blend two almonds per ounce of water at high speed. You now have a sugar- and dairy-free protein-rich drink that you can use as a base to add your protein powder to or get creative with. Almond milk will keep, if refrigerated, for several days.

ALMOND CHAI

1 cup almond milk

¼ teaspoon crushed cardamom seeds (make sure that once you remove the outer green pod, they are a dark color and aromatic)

¼ teaspoon ground cinnamon

Pinch freshly grated nutmeg

Pinch ground cloves

Tiny pinch freshly ground black pepper

1-inch piece fresh ginger, peeled and grated or sliced thinly

1 scoop protein powder

Blend in the blender until smooth and creamy.

SOY DREAM

> 1 cup fresh soy milk (refrigerated kind, not the "boxes" in the grocery section)
> ¼ teaspoon vanilla extract
> 1 scoop protein powder

Blend in the blender.

You can mix and match any variation of soy and almond milk. For those who include dairy in their diet, low-fat milk, yogurt, or kefir will blend nicely and make an excellent protein drink.

HOW TO SURVIVE THE DAY

Now, on to the rest of the day: You should eat again about two to three hours after your protein drink or smoothie. If this turns out to be a fifteen-minute morning break at work, two hard-boiled eggs pack well and are quick enough. If you long for a piece of bread, buy the sprouted type and have *one* piece, now and again, rather than daily or throughout the day. Try spreading tahini or almond or peanut butter on it instead of butter and jam. A sprouted tortilla with almond butter makes a good little meal as well. Tempeh or turkey bacon is an excellent source of protein.

Perhaps you and a group of friends go to brunch, and as you eye all the choices the menu has to offer, you find a few temptations. Remember, you always make the choice of what you eat. As you work with this new way of eating, the foods that previously attracted you may become less and less tempting. Focus on what you feel you need in the moment instead of what your friends may order. If you crave sugar, you need protein. If you crave breads, pasta, rice, pastry, cakes, pies, cookies, and ice cream, eat protein first and see if your cravings subside. Eat more slowly and chew your food thoughtfully.

Drink at least one liter or more of pure water throughout each day to help flush out toxins. Toxins inflate fat cells. As we cleanse toxins from our bodies, our internal organs function better and it is easier to lose excess weight.

SAMPLE MENUS FOR YOU TO TRY

BREAKFAST
I. Tea/coffee without sugar
Eggs (any style but fried)
Small glass of juice
(no added sugar)

II. Tea/coffee without sugar
and/or protein drink

MIDMORNING MEAL
I. Protein drink

II. Two slices of sautéed tofu

LUNCH
I. Broiled fish
Salad with oil and vinegar
dressing
½ orange, sliced

II. Baked polenta
Steamed veggies with light
butter, lemon, and herb sauce

MIDAFTERNOON MEAL
I. Apple slices with cheese

II. Sprouted tortilla and nut
butter

DINNER
I. Cup of soup (not cream-based)
Small baked potato (no dairy
toppings)
Grilled or baked turkey
tenderloin
Green beans tossed with herbs

II. Salad with oil and vinegar
Marinated tempeh, sautéed
Steamed potato
Steamed veggies in a low-fat or
fat-free sauce

AFTER DINNER
Relax with your favorite herbal tea. An occasional glass of wine or any of your favorite beverages is fine. But if you are having hot flashes and night sweats, alcohol will make them much worse and increase their frequency.

If you really want to munch on something, and you run on the hot side, try slices of raw jicama, cucumber, or celery. These vegetables are cool, crunchy, and don't add calories.

HOMEOPATHIC REMEDIES

There are many different homeopathic remedies to support the body and encourage balance of the constitution. The following remedies correlate with excessive weight and can be useful to augment the process of weight loss while you balance your hormones and change your eating habits. If you know your constitutional remedy, take it when you become out of balance as your first line of restoration.

- *Antimonium Crudum* for the woman who loves food and loves to eat, often craving sour foods like pickles, which cause digestive disturbances such as diarrhea or alternating diarrhea and constipation.
- *Calcarea Carbonica* for the woman who craves sweets, pastries, ice cream, milk, and cheeses, as well as salty foods, all of which disturb her digestion and plague her with constipation.
- *Carbo Vegetabilis* for women who often present with weak digestion, distension, and bloating and tend to long for sweets and salty foods. These women may seem unresponsive to food altogether or, conversely, approach food with voracity.
- *Ferrum* for the woman who desires sweets, bread, and butter; feeling insatiable or uninterested in food, she may experience abdominal pains when repositioning herself.
- *Graphites* for the woman who tends toward constipation and prefers blander, simple foods—chicken, beer, and sometimes sweets.
- *Kali Bichromicum* for the woman who yearns for sweets and leans toward diarrhea or colitis.
- *Kali Carbonicum* for the woman who loves sweets and becomes constipated just prior to or with her menses.
- *Lycopodium* for the woman who has many digestive disturbances, though she enjoys sweets and has an insatiable appetite.
- *Pulsatilla* for the woman who loves to eat butter, cheeses, creamy foods, and sweets, though rich and fatty foods cause her indigestion.

HERBAL FORMULAS

There are many natural herbal formulas on the market, so many that it can be overwhelming to know how to choose. Avoid those that promise you a quick fix or that you'll lose ten pounds in forty-eight hours. Often these formulas have a diuretic principle, force-flushing your kidneys, resulting in profuse urination and false hope. The weight loss is actually fluid loss and rarely addresses actual excess body fat. Some of these formulas tell you not to eat during the first two days of taking their product. While you fast, it can feel like weight loss. But as soon as you resume normal eating, not only does the weight return, you often gain more weight because your body thought you were starving and compensates.

Many formulas fall into a category I refer to as Band-Aid therapy, which means that they offer only temporary relief. Short-term treatments do sometimes act as a catalyst to initiate positive change, help reduce superficial concerns, and give you the opportunity to address deeper issues. But if you rely on repeated short-term treatments, you can do yourself harm. No formula resolves the issue of weight gain completely if your hormones remain unbalanced and your diet needs serious work. Thoroughly investigate a formula before investing your money, your trust, and your health to it. Choose one that nourishes you while you reestablish healthy eating habits.

CHINESE HERBAL FORMULAS

These formulas support weight loss while they nourish the systems. Any Chinese herbs are best taken under the direction of your herbalist or practitioner.

- *Ginseng and Astragalus Formula*
- *Ginseng Nourishing Formula*
- *Salvia Ten Formula*

MOVING YOUR BODY AND ENJOYING IT

In order for an exercise regime to be effective, you need to do two things: You must enjoy it and you must be consistent with it, a minimum of three times a week. Do you hate to exercise? Is it because you have gotten so out of shape that either you believe it's hopeless or you're too embarrassed to go to a class? Is it finances—you can't afford a class at this time? When we get stuck in any mind-set, and believe that we cannot do it, then, truly, it is impossible to succeed at whatever it is. When you focus on what does not work in your life, nothing seems to flow smoothly. Conversely, if you focus on what *is* working in your life, you will find yourself in the flow. Moving your body moves your energy and shifts your focus onto the positive and what is working. Energy moves to the rhythm of the mind. The "law of similars," the idea that like attracts like, extends into any aspect of life. We become like magnets for whatever energy or state of mind we sustain in any given moment. And as we alter the mind through exercise to a more positive state of consciousness, we then also change what we attract into our lives.

If money is your obstacle to exercise, you can commit to taking a walk. You can walk anywhere you feel safe, whether it is a walk to work or a walk around your neighborhood. For many years I had practiced yoga, even taught it. Yet I hardly noticed when I stopped doing my daily practice and slipped into a work pattern devoid of much bodily movement. As you may suspect, my energy declined into a less perky experience and I gathered more fluff in the places I wanted it the least.

A friend told me about an energy-training program she practiced that she felt had changed her life in many ways. I had been one of those women who hate going to an exercise class. I practiced yoga at home, alone. But I became lazy when it came to exercise, and a bit bored doing it alone. So I went to the Dahn Center to check out my friend's class. Not only did I come away pleasantly surprised, but energized as well. This particular practice, Dahn Hak, is a combination of aerobic yoga, chi gong, and tai chi put to music. For more information on Dahn Hak, go to *www.healingsociety.org/mair.html.*

Find a form of movement that makes you happy. If it's drudgery, any attempt at consistency becomes another piece of work to accomplish. What movement makes you smile and laugh? Is it dance? Put on the music that stirs your spirit and makes your body move, no matter how much you resist it. When you are home alone, notice where you have a negative focus. Is it your abdomen? Try patting your belly and saying out loud "I love my stomach," and smile when you do it. Let yourself have a little fun and get playful with yourself. Let your hands move where they will, to the places you may dream of changing. Instead of focusing on how much fat jiggles when you touch it, pat your butt, thighs, or knees and say "I love my butt, I love my thighs, I love my knees." Say it with enthusiasm in your voice. Don't censure your volume, and say it more than once. Remember how often you may have said the opposite to yourself. It is time to create new patterns, to dissolve the old paradigm of hating who and what we are, to turn away from the desire to look like the pictures society continues to support.

RX SUMMARY FOR HORMONAL IMBALANCE AND WEIGHT GAIN

1. Evaluate your current hormonal condition.
2. Compounded phytogenic hormone therapy, taken twice a day:

   - Biestrogen/triestrogen and progesterone (plus DHEA/testosterone) based on your hormonal analysis or symptoms
   - Find the optimal balance for you right now, and understand that your formula is likely to change in order to maintain your balance.
   - Tell your prescribing practitioner when you begin to notice a shift in your balance. She or he will not know if there is a need to change your formula unless you communicate any changes in your symptoms. Refer to the Hormonal Checklist on page 41.

In addition to phytogenic hormone therapy, you may want to consider augmentation by doing the following:

3. Change your eating habits.

   - Eat small, frequent meals.
   - Eat a whole-foods diet: Read labels before you buy, and choose foods
       Low in sugar
       Low in carbohydrates
       Low in fat
       High in protein
       High in fiber
   - Avoid commercially raised meats and dairy containing exogenous hormones, antibiotics, pesticides, and unnecessary chemicals.
   - Avoid *all* refined, processed foods.

- Minimize caffeine and alcohol.
- Use stevia instead of sugar as your sweetener.
- Don't eat late at night. Try not to eat later than four hours before bedtime.
- Don't eat to alleviate stress—find other outlets.
- Don't eat comfort foods.
- Add low-calorie/low-carbohydrate protein drinks to your diet.
- Eat veggies such as jicama, celery, and cucumbers as snacks instead of chips and pretzels.

4. Rule out thyroid dysfunction and adrenal exhaustion.
5. Homeopathic assistance

   - Antimonium Crudum
   - Calcarea Carbonica
   - Carbo Vegetabilis
   - Ferrum
   - Graphites
   - Kali Bichromicum
   - Kali Carbonicum
   - Lycopodium
   - Pulsatilla

6. Chinese Herbal Support

   - Ginseng and Astragalus Formula
   - Ginseng Nourishing Formula
   - Salvia Ten Formula

7. Balanced multivitamins and minerals
8. Pay attention to your stress level/management.
9. Nurture yourself with kindness, forgiveness, and compassion.
10. Acupuncture
11. Find a way of moving your body that works for you and do it consistently.

THYROID DYSFUNCTION WITH HORMONAL WEIGHT GAIN

Hypothyroidism, an underactive thyroid condition, is the most common thyroid dysfunction accompanying the menopausal process or hormonal imbalances. (Please refer to Chapter 2, page 28, for more information on the thyroid.)

Tricia, age forty-four

> I've been following this diet of eating small, frequent meals for three months now. I'm not gaining more weight, but I'm not losing any either. When I crave sweets, I'm eating protein instead. I've been trying to exercise. But I'm so tired most of the time, I kind of feel depressed because I just don't have enough energy to do things that are important to me. Thank God my kids don't need much from me, now that they're grown up. Since I've been taking the natural hormones I'm not getting hot flashes anymore, but now I'm tending to be cold. What's wrong with me?

At forty-four years of age, Tricia did not think she was going into menopause. Her hormonal analysis showed her progesterone was consistently below normal through day twenty-one, peaked for two days, and then dropped below normal again. The DHEA measured below normal, her estrogens were in the low range of normal, and her testosterone was in the middle of the normal range.

Initially she felt better after taking a formula tailored for not only the results of the hormonal analysis but her symptoms as well. Tricia took progesterone throughout her cycle (beginning with 35 mg for the first week, increasing to 50 mg on days thirteen through eighteen, 100 mg on days nineteen through twenty-four, then back to 50 mg) until she began to bleed, during which she took nothing. She takes her progesterone in an oral capsule and 1 mg of DHEA as a drop under her tongue, which she can increase according to her energy level. Her formula resolved her insomnia, hot flashes and night sweats, breast pain, increased anxiety, and irritability within one month. With the hormones causing her menopausal symptoms balanced, her stressed thyroid reared itself for attention.

Often, perimenopausal and menopausal women discover that their thyroid is functioning poorly. We must consider all hormonal functions as we reestablish balance, including our thyroid and adrenals. If you find yourself continuing to gain weight when you are on a balanced compounded phytogenic hormonal formula, and you have a good diet with a consistently regular exercise program, test your thyroid.

Thyroid dysfunctions can be missed on a routine blood test. I prefer the salivary test to evaluate the thyroid because it reveals more information for me to consider, and at a lower cost to the woman. Most serum thyroid tests, taken through a blood sample, focus on thyroid stimulating hormone (TSH), and if that is elevated, the lab then measures L-thyroxine (T4). For as long as I've been in practice, I've observed many women who have been symptomatic of hypothyroidism, an underactive thyroid, but with normal serum analysis. If the woman is left untreated and her thyroid does not correct the imbalance spontaneously, a serum analysis will eventually show abnormal levels. The salivary analysis, however, seems to reveal below normal levels sooner than the serum test, and it correlates more closely with a woman's experience.

Tricia's salivary thyroid analysis revealed an elevated TSH, an extremely low T4, and low triiodothyronine (T3). For Tricia to fully restore balance, she needed to supplement with a thyroid formula as well. One such natural option is an inexpensive form called Bio-Throid, available through the Women's International Pharmacy. Packed into a small capsule, Bio-Throid's T3 and T4 is an extracted porcine glandular hormone and does not contain corn or additives to which one may have allergic reactions. How long Tricia will continue to supplement at one grain daily remains unclear at the time of this writing. It is possible for her thyroid to reestablish normal functioning through short-term therapy.

Tammy, age forty-six

Tammy, on the other hand, complained of her hair falling out by the handful. Her relentless weight instability, regardless of her unswerving exercise regime, caused her much despair. The return of terrible sleep disturbances and insomnia left her so exhausted that she could barely see straight. We had addressed her adrenal exhaustion several months earlier, and her hormonal formula of 2.5 mg of biestrogen, 100 mg of progesterone, and 5 mg of DHEA, taken in the morning, with a higher dose of estrogen at bedtime, served her well with her menopausal symptoms.

I'm not exactly fat. When I tell friends that I want to lose this extra weight, they roll their eyes at me. My diet's good, and I've cut down on the amounts I'm eating, but I've not lost one single pound, not one inch. And I know the difference between fat and muscle. It's so frustrating that I just want to give up, eat a pound of chocolate, and watch TV. My energy is okay, but I still need a nap every day.

The values of Tammy's serum thyroid analysis were normal. And all the values on the salivary test were normal as well, except for her T3, which was quite below normal. She began supplementing with 15 mcg of T3, for a trial period, with the intention of stimulating her thyroid back into functioning at its optimum. She then tried the Bio-Throid formula, which seemed to support her energy level and weight loss better.

In the case of both of these women, estrogen dominance was not the cause of their hypothyroidism. Their perimenopausal symptoms were addressed first, and as you can see, they take very different hormonal formulas. Their thyroid testing was not done until after their other hormonal imbalances had been identified and supported, and their disturbing menopausal symptoms resolved.

NATURAL TREATMENT OPTIONS

Compounded Phytogenic Natural Hormones

Evaluate your hormones and begin a formula to restore your general hormonal balance. When you test with the salivary or twenty-four-hour urine analysis, measure all your hormones (including thyroid) and your cortisol levels.

The dosage of your formula will depend on how deficient you are based on these levels, as well as your symptoms.

Desiccated Thyroid Glandulars

Rx: *Bio-Throid,* by Bio-Tech, is a natural desiccated thyroid from a porcine source, with the same ratio of T3 and T4 as Armor Thyroid but without the fillers and other substances, such as corn, to which some people are allergic and which those with candidiasis function better without. It comes in as low a dosage as one-quarter grain, or can be filled in one- or two-grain capsules. I like it better than Armor because the dosage seems to distribute a more evenly consistent potency, and it does not have a stinky odor. Women's International Pharmacy carries Bio-Throid in all its available potencies.

Nature-Throid, by Western Research Laboratories, is also from a porcine source, identical to Westhroid, developed in 1934, except that it does not contain cornstarch.

OTC: Different companies manufacture glandular compounds, some of which are extracted from a bovine source (cow) instead of porcine (pig). Companies such as Tyler, in their formula called *BMR,* and Allergy Research Group, in its TG100, utilize resources from free-range New Zealand cows that are not pumped full of pesticides, hormones, or antibiotics. Although their integrity is admirable, due to FDA regulations, the amount of actual thyroid contained in each capsule is significantly low. This means that someone with a serious thyroid condition must take many capsules to accomplish a close-to-adequate dosage.

Other formulas, such as *Tyrosine Complex,* contain B-12, iodine, magnesium, zinc, manganese, L-tyrosine, multiglandular complex, and thyroxine-free thyroid substance.

OTHER NATURAL THYROID SUPPORT OPTIONS

Homeopathic Remedies
- *Apo-Strum* is indicated for treatment of thyroid dysfunctions including hardening or enlargement of the thyroid gland.
- *Calcarea Carbonica* can support hypothyroidism in someone who tends to be chilly and get cold easily, while also easily gaining weight.
- *Kali Iodatum* assists with both hypothyroidism and hyperthyroidism, with or without the presence of a goiter.

Herbal Nutritionals
Thyroid Support includes bladder wrack, collinsonia, coleus, kelp, and L-tyrosine, and is available at: *www.gaiaherbs.com/products/newphytos/ css/thyroidsupport.*

An Ayurvedic thyroid medicine called *Ashwagandha* (*Withania Sominifera*), also known as Indian ginseng, states that it increases thyroxine and T3.

Chinese Herbal Supports
- *Ginseng and Astragalus Formula*
- *Ginseng Nourishing Formula*

For more information on the next two formulas, go to *www.herb-doc.com/thyroid.htm*.

- Thyro-H#450 assists in hyperthyroidism.
- Thyro-H#455 assists in hypothyroidism.

Dietary Considerations
Certain foods, such as vegetables in the crucifer family—cabbages, cresses, mustard greens, cauliflower, broccoli—actually increase thyroxine levels. Seaweeds, especially kelp, due to their high iodine content, are supportive in hypothyroidism. Tea made from either walnuts or butternuts can also increase thyroxine.

For hyperthyroid conditions, herbs such as verbena, lemon balm, and bugleweed have been shown to exhibit hypoactive qualities, which may help slow down the hyperactive thyroid.

Vitamin Support
Specific vitamins assist in the production of thyroid hormone. These include vitamins A, E, C, niacin, pyridoxine, and riboflavin.

RX SUMMARY FOR HYPOTHYROIDISM WITH HORMONAL WEIGHT GAIN

1. Test your thyroid.

- Measure your *basal temperature* before rising, and three to four times a day for three to six days (use the chart on page 32). If your temperature measures at a consistently low level of 97.8°F or less for one week, then:
- Do a salivary or twenty-four-hour urine thyroid analysis.

2. Compounded phytogenic hormone therapy, taken twice a day:

   - Biestrogen/triestrogen, progesterone (DHEA/testosterone): based on your hormonal analysis or symptoms
   - Find the optimal balance for you right now, and understand that your formula is likely to change in order to maintain your balance.
   - In addition to phytogenic hormone therapy, you will need thyroid medication; consider augmentation with:

3. Natural thyroid treatment options:

   - Natural thyroid Rx, dosage based on testing, often beginning as low as ¼ gr
     Bio-Throid
     Nature-Throid

   - Other natural thyroid support, which may be less potent
     *Natural glandular formulas, OTC: BMR, TG100, Tyrosine
        Complex*
     Ashwagandha, Indian ginseng
     Homeopathy: Apo-Strum, Calcarea Carbonica, Kali Iodatum
     *Herbal support: Ginseng and Astragalus Formula, Ginseng
        Nourishing Formula, Thyro-H#450, Thyro-H#455*
     *Follow the diet recommendations to avoid weight gain, described
        earlier in this chapter, with the addition of: cruciferous vegetables,
        kelp and other seaweeds, and walnut or butternut tea.*

4. Balanced multivitamins, minerals, and antioxidants, with adequate B-12, and including:

   - Vitamin A (25,000 IU)
   - Vitamin C (1,000 mg or up to bowel tolerance)
   - Vitamin E (400 IU)
   - Niacin (50 mg)
   - Pyridoxine (50 mg)
   - Riboflavin (15 mg)
   - Zinc (30 mg)

- Iodine (300 mcg)
- Tyrosine (250–500 mg twice a day)

5. Rule out adrenal exhaustion by salivary or urine analysis.
6. Slow down, discover your rhythm.
7. Take naps if you need to until your thyroid and hormones establish a reliable balance.
8. Incorporate exercise that you can handle—walking, swimming, yoga, tai chi.

ADRENAL EXHAUSTION

The expression "burning the candle at both ends" describes quite accurately how a woman feels when she experiences adrenal exhaustion.

Caffeine intake increases our adrenaline levels; with continued heavy caffeine use, the adrenal glands can be pushed to the point of inability to release ample adrenaline in response to stress. Adrenal exhaustion rapidly ensues. Adrenal exhaustion often alters hormonal balance because the ability of the innermost layer of the adrenal gland, the zona reticularis, to produce estrogens, progesterone, and androgen hormones is compromised. Although it is possible to have difficulty gaining weight with this condition, more commonly it seems to support weight gain.

Possible Causes of Adrenal Stress Leading to Adrenal Exhaustion
- Continually overworked and overburdened
- Prolonged physical and/or mental strain
- Excessive exercise
- Sleep deprivation
- Interruption of normal light cycles
- Nutritional deficiencies, malabsorption, poor digestion, hypoglycemia
- External stresses: trauma, injury, surgery, toxic exposure, exposure to temperature extremes
- Chronic conditions of illness, infection, inflammation, pain, and allergies
- Chronic or sustained heightened emotional states: anger, fear, worry, depression, anxiety, guilt

NATURAL TREATMENT OPTIONS

Compounded Phytogenic Natural Hormones

Evaluate your hormones and begin a formula to restore your general hormonal balance. Commonly, when one is in adrenal exhaustion, the DHEA is deficient because our adrenal glands provide the most abundant source of DHEA, secreting greater quantities of it than of any other adrenal steroid. When you test with the salivary or twenty-four-hour urine analysis, also measure your cortisol levels and thyroid hormones.

The dosage of your formula will depend on how deficient you are based on these levels as well as your symptoms. It is common for a woman in adrenal exhaustion to need as much as 50 mg of DHEA daily, best taken in the morning. The quality of DHEA and how you take it will affect absorption, utilization, and how quickly you recover. Remember, if you experience digestive disturbances, you may better absorb your hormones by taking them either under your tongue or by application to your skin.

Adrenal Glandulars
- Whole, desiccated adrenal extract
- ACE, adrenocortico extracts

Homeopathic Remedies

Consider your constitutional remedy or one of the following combination remedies.

These formulas, produced by Heel, Inc., suggest the average dosage as 10 drops taken orally three times a day. For more information on Heel and BHI, go to *www.heelbhi.com*.

- *Aletris-Heel* relieves symptoms of exhaustion and weakness following overexertion.
- *China-Homaccord* helps with the relief of fatigue and exhaustion caused by stress, overwork, and chronic illness.
- *Galium-Heel* assists in increasing the activation of the body's defense mechanisms.
- *Nervoheel* relieves symptoms of stress, restlessness, insomnia, and nervous tension.

- *Selenium-Homaccord* assists with stress-related mental fatigue and the inability to concentrate.
- *Ypsiloheel* works for stress and nervous irritability.
- *BHI Exhaustion* aids in relief of fatigue and exhaustion following exertion, overwork, stress, insomnia, and is useful during or following illness.

Herbal Support

Many Chinese herbal formulas that include astragalus, licorice, and/or ginseng can be beneficial. Much depends on the specific combinations of your symptoms, which would be best assessed and formulated by your practitioner.

- Licorice root
- Panax ginseng and Siberian ginseng

Additional Vitamins and Minerals

Vitamin B-15 (pangamic acid) helps regulate the hypothalamus, pituitary, and adrenal axis. It also eliminates jet lag. Other vitamins essential for proper adrenal gland function include: vitamin B-5 (pantothenic acid), vitamin B-6 (pyridoxine), vitamin C with bioflavonoids, vitamin E, PABA, potassium, magnesium, and zinc.

Other Nutrients

- *Trimethylglycine (TMG)* helps the adrenal gland maintain function and produce hormones.
- *Antioxidants* such as coenzyme Q10, alpha-lipoic acid, and methyl-sulfonylmethane (MSM) promote cellular health.

RX SUMMARY FOR ADRENAL EXHAUSTION

1. Rule out hormone imbalances, DHEA deficiency, and thyroid dysfunction.
2. Compounded phytogenic hormone formula, including DHEA, taken twice a day, tailored specifically to your needs
3. Test your adrenal function through salivary or twenty-four-hour urine analysis.

In addition to phytogenic hormone therapy, you will need adrenal medicines and support; consider augmentation with:

4. Natural adrenal support

   - Adrenal glandulars—whole, desiccated adrenal gland extract
   - Homeopathy
       Constitutional remedy, or single remedy
       Aletris-Heel
       China-Homaccord
       Galium-Heel
       Nervoheel
       Selenium-Homaccord
       Ypsiloheel
       BHI Exhaustion

   - Herbal support
       Licorice Root
       Panax Ginseng
       Siberian Ginseng

   - Vitamins, minerals, and antioxidants
   - Other nutrients
       Coenzyme Q10
       Alpha-lipoic Acid
       MSM
       TMG

5. Dietary changes to include a whole-foods diet of

   - High protein (twice the amount of protein as carbohydrate)
   - Low carbohydrates (one carbohydrate to two proteins)
   - Low sugar
   - High fiber
   - Include a small amount of fat in each meal.
   - Increase drinking pure water, 1–2 liters a day.
   - Avoid caffeine: coffee, sodas, black teas, cocoa.
   - Eat small meals often, and before you get hungry.

- Eat within one hour of awakening.
- Balance each meal to support optimal blood sugar function.

6. Eliminate or reduce stress as much as possible; refer to suggestions found in Chapters 3, 7, and 9.
7. Try meditation and/or slow, deep-breathing exercises.
8. Rest—get adequate sleep, go to bed earlier.
9. Discontinue rigorous forms of exercise that exhaust you further until you no longer suffer from adrenal exhaustion.
10. Practice regenerating forms of exercise—yoga, chi gong, tai chi.

THE FEMININE METAMORPHOSIS

PERIMENOPAUSE THROUGH POSTMENOPAUSE

WHAT IS PERIMENOPAUSE?

Our internal biorhythms, general health, and genetics influence when our hormones begin to shift and decline, and when their normal ratios become somewhat out of sync. This begins the perimenopausal phase of a woman's life, which may take up to fifteen years before she transits into postmenopause. Early signs characteristic of perimenopause can be so mild that they go unnoticed, or so extreme that a woman may feel something is terribly wrong with her. Often progesterone is the primary hormone that becomes the most deficient. But DHEA, the estrogens, and testosterone may also become deficient at this stage.

Compounded phytogenic natural hormones ameliorate the physical and psychological symptoms by addressing the underlying cause of hormonal deficiencies. This commonly requires a process of fine-tuning, making adjustments in the dosage of hormones put into your formula, as well as changing the specific hormones you need to augment. Occasionally, some women require additional therapeutic measures because of the severity of their experience and the need for immediate intervention if their hormonal balance does not respond quickly enough.

Perimenopausal/Menopausal Symptoms

Sixty-six Physical Symptoms: These are very real physical changes and conditions. Some are so alarming that a woman may feel she has a serious disease. You may know the more common symptoms on this list. But others may surprise you, as they have not been typically associated with this normal life transformation.

1. *Change in menstrual cycle.* Cycles may get closer together or further apart, lighter and shorter in duration or much heavier and lasting longer than what you have been accustomed to. Menses may seem to take forever to begin, with dark spotting for days until you actually flow, or you might feel like you have your menses every two weeks.
2. *Menstrual flooding* can come on with sudden onset and you feel as if you may hemorrhage to death. Or it can be a gradual buildup just when you think your menses will end, and you start gushing for days. Flooding commonly accompanies the presence of uterine fibroids as a woman transits into menopause.
3. *Headaches or migraines,* especially before, during, or at the end of your menses, debilitate and radically interfere with normal functioning.
4. *Decreased motor coordination and clumsiness* almost begin to make a woman feel as if she is a bit spastic, and certainly less than graceful during perhaps an already awkward period in her life.
5. *Lethargy,* a persistent feeling of sluggishness—both physically and mentally—that seems to negate one's ability to do much.
6. *Physical exhaustion and crushing, crashing fatigue* that can come on so suddenly that you feel you will collapse unless you stop whatever you are doing immediately.
7. *Exacerbation of any chronic illness or existing condition* occurs as hormones decline or deviate from their normal balance.
8. *Insomnia.* This includes a new or unusual pattern of either difficulty falling asleep or dropping off to sleep for a few hours and then awakening with the inability to return to sleep.
9. *Sleep disturbances*—ranging from nightmares to night sweats to just a vague sense of restlessness—keep you up or disrupt your precious revitalizing time.

10. *Night sweats* often begin between a woman's breasts, initially a night or two before her menses, and wake her from sleep. Later, they are more profoundly disturbing, with up to total body saturation followed by damp or sweat-drenched chills.

11. *Interference with dream recall* interrupts the sense of normal sleep if you are accustomed to vivid or at least some detailed memory of your dreams.

12. *Muscle cramps* can occur anywhere in the body, from legs to back to neck, and sometimes reflect the need for more calcium, or simply that your progesterone levels are too low.

13. *Low backache* often worsens before or during menses, but if your hormones remain at low levels, you can experience it on a regular basis.

14. *Gallbladder symptoms* of pain, spasms, and discomfort felt in the right upper abdominal quadrant under the ribs, which may be accompanied by belching, bloating, and intolerance to certain foods, reflect the increased liver load with declining hormones.

15. *Frequent urination,* or sensations that mimic urinary infections, is a disturbing symptom. It is often experienced as the sensation of needing to urinate all the time, even immediately after having done so.

16. *Urinary incontinence,* the uncontrollable and spontaneous loss of urine, or the *urge for incontinence,* can occur suddenly or feel continuous, and not only in response to coughing, sneezing, jumping, or running.

17. *Hypoglycemic reactions* happen when your blood sugar suddenly crashes and you must have food *now.*

18. *Food cravings,* often for sweets or salty foods, but can include sour or pungent foods.

19. *Increased appetite,* especially at night and after dinner, contributes to unusual and unwanted weight gain.

20. *Dark circles under the eyes* that no amount of sleep seems to eliminate can also be caused by adrenal exhaustion and thyroid dysfunction.

21. *Joint and muscle pain.* Achy, sore joints, muscles, and tendons sometimes develop into actual carpal tunnel syndrome or give rise to wondering about other disease possibilities.

22. *Increased tension in muscles* demonstrates itself in hunched up

shoulders as you work or talk about anything uncomfortable, along with promoting lower back pain and a stiff neck.

23. *Increased hair loss or thinning* anywhere on the body—head, armpits, pubic area.

24. *An increase in facial hair,* especially under the chin or along the jawline, that may be defined by generalized hair growth, or a specific and coarse single strand of hair that pokes out and even curls.

25. *Unusual hair growth* around nipples, between breasts, down your back—places where your hair was finer, less coarse.

26. *Acne.* This is quite disturbing to any woman who dealt with this in adolescence and never thought it would recur.

27. *Infertility* causes grief in the woman who postponed pregnancy in her earlier years and now wishes to conceive and carry to term a healthy baby, and discovers she is unable to do so.

28. *Loss of breast tissue* begins with the decrease of progesterone production. Women often feel as though their breasts have become empty sacs devoid of their normal fullness, with or without sagging.

29. *Breast soreness/tenderness/pain/engorgement and swelling* occur particularly a few days to one week before bleeding actually begins, which usually brings complete relief of any pain or swelling.

30. *Painful or tender nipples* have been described as an exquisite, localized pain only in the nipples, which suggests estrogen excess.

31. *Cold extremities* feel quite strange, especially in the presence of a hot flash, the combination of which is not impossible.

32. *Being accident prone,* bumping into things and not even realizing it until the bruise reveals itself later and then lacking the ability to recall the causative incident, feels perplexing and a little scary at the prospect of something more serious.

33. *Hot flashes* initially may be described as mild to severe flashes of heat waves, and for some women these evolve into intense outbreaks of sudden heat with sweating and turning bright red all over.

34. *Loss of sexual energy, or libido,* can be marked by a gradual or sudden disinterest in sex or even an actual aversion to it.

35. *Painful sex,* often described as if one's vagina would tear open at the point of penetration, along with feelings of abrasion during intercourse.

36. *Vaginal dryness, irritation*, sometimes accompanied by a consistent, unusual discharge—typically odor free—negates a woman's ability to be sexually active or to enjoy or be comfortable in her body.

37. *Dizziness,* feeling lightheaded with the loss of physical balance, or even a bit wobbly at times, requires pause in movement to prevent falling over; sometimes deepens into vertigo or feeling faint.

38. *Ringing in the ears, or tinnitus,* can be experienced as a pulsing sensation, a whooshing sound, an almost musical or buzzing sound with a fuzzy sensation.

39. *Abdominal bloating* comes on suddenly, often after eating, or seems to be present all the time and can be visibly evident, making you feel that you look pregnant.

40. *Weight gain* disturbs most women, particularly when it seems to happen over a couple of days; settles in the waist, buttocks, and thighs; and promotes a visceral thickening from the waist down, the classic middle-aged figure.

41. *Fluid retention, or edema,* commonly with swelling in the legs and ankles, though not limited to this area; it is unrelieved by urination.

42. *Palpitations, or heart racing,* usually comes on suddenly, without warning or provocation, and dissipates spontaneously. The experience can be so wild and intense that a woman may become alarmed and wonder if she is having a heart attack.

43. *Irregularities in your heart rate* may feel as if your heart has just done a flip-flop or skipped a beat.

44. *Constipation/diarrhea, intermittent or alternating,* results from declining hormone levels, which increase the demands on liver function and alter intestinal motility.

45. *Tendency toward candidiasis* can increase, even if you have no prior history—and if you do, it may worsen.

46. *Gastrointestinal distress, increased flatulence, unrelieved gas pains, indigestion, and/or nausea*—all can reflect intestinal changes due to hormonal imbalances.

47. *Slow digestion* often goes along with the bloat—what previously took four to five hours to digest now seems to take all night. It may seem worse in the evenings.

48. *Lack of appetite* may be experienced as more of a lack of interest in food, going to the fridge and standing there with the door open and

staring blankly. Feeling completely uninspired, you busy yourself with something else and forget that you need to eat.

49. *Changes in body odor*—especially disturbing when it seems to focus in the groin area but can be anywhere on the body.

50. *Puffy eyes* come not only from sleep disturbances but also may accompany low progesterone.

51. *Facial pallor* alternating with *facial flushing* is often intermittent with hot flashes.

52. *Flare-up of arthritis* that worsens with low progesterone levels and increased sugar intake.

53. *Loss of bone density, or osteoporosis*, is not only an elderly woman's disease, though it seems to develop over an extended period and is triggered by the decline of hormone production, especially progesterone.

54. *Dry hair and change in skin tone, integrity, and texture* as skin becomes more wrinkled; may be the beginning of the thinning process.

55. *Changes in fingernails*, characterized by easy breakage, bending, cracking, and softening.

56. *Itchy, crawly skin* with a strange sensation like insects crawling around under the skin—quite different from the dry-skin feeling.

57. *Muscle tone* seems to be slack and sagging; muscles lose their previous response to normal exercise.

58. *Pelvic pain* can be random and independent of cycles and may feel continuous for some women.

59. *Dry, itchy eyes* felt in the deep posterior aspect of the eye socket, as well as superficially.

60. *Teeth aching* or the experience of a strange sensation in one's teeth or gums, often accompanied by an increase in bleeding gums.

61. *Change in normal tongue sensation*, which can be accompanied by a feeling of burning in your tongue and the roof of your mouth, malodorous breath or change in breath odor, and/or a bad taste in your mouth.

62. *Memory loss or lapses in time* make you feel disoriented and less focused, especially when you go into another room to get something specific and seconds later cannot remember what you went to retrieve.

63. *Feeling faint* for no known reason (this does not include standing up too quickly).

64. *Tingling in extremities* not only feels weird and as if your hands or feet are falling asleep, but if persistent can be a symptom of diabetes; B-12, potassium, or calcium deficiency; or a compromise in blood vessel flexibility.

65. *Sensation of electrical stimulation, prick, or shock* occurring in the tissue under the skin, which may be a signal that a hot flash will begin.

66. *Increase and worsening of allergies.* Just as hormones become imbalanced, so can the immune system.

Twenty-five Psychological and Emotional Symptoms: You may feel as if you've stepped onto the emotional roller-coaster ride of your life without ever giving your conscious consent to the ride. The emotional aspects can be intense, often described like feeling stuck in a relentless PMS loop with all the perceptible alterations suffered to an extreme. Most of these symptoms are a result of progesterone deficiency and can be relieved with natural progesterone alone. Some, such as numbers 2, 9, 11, and 12, may require the addition of estrogens and/or DHEA. Others, if unresolved with phytogenic hormones, may necessitate intervention and/or alternate therapy.

1. *Crying or weeping spontaneously,* which may be uncontrollable and either exaggerated for the circumstance, inappropriate, or unprovoked.

2. *Feelings of panic,* usually without warning and beyond one's control to change, which may be accompanied by heart palpitations or a racing sensation.

3. *Feeling easily frustrated* and having a *very short fuse* can lead to hasty and sometimes inappropriate reactions and/or decisions, not to mention glass breakage.

4. *Feeling violent, aggressive, or hostile* may or may not be expressed, and when this remains suppressed or inappropriately expressed repeatedly over time, serious disturbances may result.

5. *Feeling self-abusive or inflicting injuries upon oneself* requires immediate attention and treatment.

6. *Sudden anger and angry outbursts,* with greater intensity than a situation may warrant, or completely unprovoked by any known

external cause, disturb one's sense of harmony or induce feelings of elation and self-satisfaction.

7. *Feelings of anxiety or terror,* often unexplained or irrational when unprovoked by outside forces, feel extremely disconcerting and if sustained can lead to a breakdown.

8. *Verbal and/or physical abuse* may flare up suddenly and be directed at anyone within range.

9. *Feelings of dread and/or apprehension,* when sustained over time, feel like a relentless weight that catalyzes disturbing behavioral changes.

10. *Loss of feeling normal or a general sense of well-being, and feeling a loss of self* can make one feel disconnected to the fabric of existence and the meaning of everyday life.

11. *Disturbing memory lapses* can be physiologic in origin or emotionally rooted. They usually respond over time to hormone therapy, unless due to organic brain disease or brain trauma.

12. *Inability to focus or concentrate, disorientation, and mental confusion* contribute to feeling abnormal and disrupt any focused, reflective activities.

13. *Irritability* is often a response to the heightened sensitivities that escort us through this transitional time, and everything from your mood to your skin may feel irritable.

14. *Mental exhaustion* and the feeling that everything is too overwhelming to consider, and even simple tasks or answering the phone becomes an effort.

15. *Depression,* often described as different from other experiences with depression, seems to well up from deep within the soul, a prolonged dark night.

16. *Feelings of hopelessness*—you're devoid of any sense of inspiration to go on with life, though not suicidal. These feelings reinforce the lethargy so often experienced in the menopausal process.

17. *Mood swings,* crying over nothing in particular one minute, feeling elated the next, and raging the one after that—the ultimate emotional antithesis of yin/yang, leading to number 18.

18. *Feelings of being crazy* happen when we cease to recognize ourselves because of all the wild, uncontrollable, physical, emotional, mental, and possibly spiritual changes we endure.

19. *Inexplicable thoughts of doom* may be so severe that one becomes fixated on one's own death, imagining the details. Effective assistance is often just a natural hormone away.

20. *Feeling suicidal or actually attempting suicide* necessitates immediate psychological and/or medical intervention.

21. *Feeling withdrawn*—curling up in a ball on the couch or under the covers works briefly but really interferes with any sense of normal everyday life. Balancing alone time and hormones transforms perception and seems to expand horizons.

22. *Feeling hysterical or actual hysteria,* beyond alternating crying jags with episodes of laughter, without provocation, can also include somatic symptoms emulating any type of physical disease. The term stems from the Greek word *hystera,* which means uterus.

23. *Feeling that anything happening is far worse* than it may be in reality, a distortion of perception, may evolve into paranoia if left unattended.

24. *Excessive use of alcohol, drugs, or other escape mechanisms,* if prolonged beyond hormonal adjustments, becomes a symptom that requires further investigation and treatment.

25. *Feeling as if you're in an existential or spiritual crisis or at a crossroads* when nothing in your life truly makes sense anymore and you know you must change your life because you simply cannot go on living like this, even if the clarity with which to accomplish this eludes you.

WHAT IS MENOPAUSE?

The transition zone between perimenopause and postmenopause is menopause. This process is our metamorphic evolutionary journey into who we are becoming for the rest of our lifetime, and often mirrors our experience of coming into puberty. We began our journey into womanhood with the onset of menarche in puberty, our first menstrual cycle. We then entered the much longer second cycle, which includes our childbearing years through menopause. Our third primary life cycle begins once we are postmenopausal.

This natural process, also a three-phase cycle, is signaled by the cessation of ovulation, as the ovarian supply of follicles and eggs declines and eventually estrogen and progesterone are no longer produced. As hormone levels drop, the lining of the uterus thins and the monthly bleeding ends. Although ovulation ends, the ovaries continue to produce some estrogen and androgen hormones.

WHAT IS POSTMENOPAUSE?

Once a woman no longer bleeds cyclically for twelve consecutive months, she is considered postmenopausal retrospectively. This does not mean she has shriveled up and become an ancient crone. For decades, advertisements have deceived us into believing a postmenopausal woman is a hunched-over old woman approaching her deathbed. This is simply not true.

Age is one factor, with onset generally occurring between the mid-forties and mid-fifties. However, I have worked with women as young as thirty-seven who were postmenopausal. Indeed, one woman I know became postmenopausal at thirty-three because of an intense trauma that induced premature menopause. Conversely, I know women who are fifty-eight years of age and continue to have regular naturally occurring menstrual cycles. This does not include all the women who, even into their eighties, bleed each month with induced false cycles due to synthetic hormone replacement therapy.

WHAT IS SURGICAL MENOPAUSE?

When a woman's uterus, both ovaries, and fallopian tubes are surgically removed—a total hysterectomy—she undergoes immediate passage into menopause, regardless of her age or the reason for the surgery. Surgical removal of both ovaries instigates the menopausal process due to the immediate cessation of the hormone production normally performed by the ovaries. Surgical removal of the uterus with the preservation of at least one ovary does not negate the production of hormones by our ovaries and therefore does not initiate the menopausal process.

Hysterectomies can sometimes be necessary and life-saving. If you are facing an inescapable hysterectomy, talk to your surgeon. Inquire about the possibility of keeping your cervix and your ovaries if you are not already postmenopausal. Your cervix plays an important role in the female orgasm, and although its removal may not negate your ability to be orgasmic, the quality of orgasms may change dramatically. Many hysterectomies are avoidable by establishing and maintaining adequate hormonal balance.

Hysterectomies Avoidable by Hormonal Management and Other Natural Modalities

- *Anovulatory bleeding,* bleeding that occurs during the time of ovulation without the production and discharge of an ovum
- *Cystocele,* the protrusion of the bladder into the vagina
- *Endometriosis,* growth of endometrial tissue outside the uterine lining
- *Dysfunctional uterine bleeding* (DUB), any uterine bleeding other than that of the normal menstrual cycle without an identified specific, organic etiology
- *Menorrhagia,* excessive bleeding at the time of a menstrual period, which may cause uterine hemorrhage
- *Rectocele,* the protrusion of the rectum into the vagina
- *Uterine fibroids,* benign uterine growths or tumors
- *Uterine prolapse,* which occurs when the uterus descends into the pelvis due to weakened support. This is most reversible in the early stage of a first-degree prolapse as the cervix moves down toward the introitus, becoming visible but not protruding outside the vagina.

Unavoidable Hysterectomies

- *Invasive carcinoma* of the cervix, endometrium, uterus, or ovaries
- *Accident or trauma* that causes severe damage or irreparable rupture to the uterus
- Any of the conditions listed above under avoidable hysterectomies that are sustained over time and become a compromise to a woman's health

Hormone management with compounded phytogenic natural hormones accomplishes the same relief for the woman who has experienced surgical menopause as for one who undergoes a natural menopausal process. Previously, women who had hysterectomies were given only estrogen, based on the assumption that they did not need progesterone because they no longer had a uterus. This practice was established when only the synthetic estrogens and progestins were prescribed. Natural progesterone continues to have necessary and beneficial functions, as described in earlier chapters, such as assisting in the prevention and treatment of osteoporosis.

WHAT ELSE INDUCES PREMATURE MENOPAUSE?

These other scenarios are less common and sometimes can be reversed if addressed early. In some women, the hormones are already out of balance, although they may not have been symptomatic enough to have had any indication.

- An intense and sudden trauma such as an automobile accident can initiate such an extreme hormonal imbalance that menopause ensues.
- A powerful and unexpected stress that pushes the woman over the top can shut down normal hormonal production.
- An abrupt and severe grief that penetrates so deeply that a woman loses herself in her loss can bring her menses to a halt.
- Exposure to toxins or radiation, by whatever means, can bring on premature menopause.
- Prolonged malnutrition, or an acute and debilitating illness may bring on the cessation of menses in the body's attempt to preserve energy.
- Some women who bear a child in their late thirties or early forties never see another menses after the one prior to conception.

The women in the following stories have multiple symptoms, but the focus is on one thing that disturbs them the most. Rarely have I seen a woman who experiences only one disconcerting menopausal symptom. Yet when this happens, that one specific concern can become so magnified that she has difficulty focusing on anything else.

It is my intention to ensure that you clearly understand how your hormones continue to fluctuate, how they can increase through stimulation with phytogenic hormones, and how they will decrease with the passage of time. Hormone formulas need to change as you progress through your metamorphosis. So you need to become an acute observer and investigator of yourself and your experiences. See what these changes evoke in you.

THE M & M BLUES

Change in cycles—closer together . . . further apart . . . heavier . . . lighter . . . skipping them altogether—what is a woman to do? It can be very disturbing for a woman to either skip her menses or bleed every other week. And it often takes adjusting her hormones several times to reestablish a more predictable pattern, which is especially important if she wants to become pregnant. Eventually all women stop bleeding—it is our destiny. But because phytogenic hormones will stimulate the production of our own hormones, some women actually restart their menses long after they thought they were finished bleeding forever.

This is not abnormal, nor is it a sign of endometrial or uterine cancer, if the return of regular menstrual cycles is in direct response to initiating compounded phytogenic natural hormones or changing to a new formula.

LATE AND NOT PREGNANT?

Lily's experience, age forty-eight

> This is a first. The only time I've ever been late for my period was when I was pregnant. I know I'm not pregnant. My cycle began to change several months ago when I changed our mattress, though I don't know if that had anything to do with it. It seems like I'm warmer than I used to be. But for me, it's a nice change because I tend to be cold. I know I must be getting closer to menopause; I'm forty-eight now. So I expect my periods to be different. What disturbs me the most is the insomnia I've developed. I fall asleep okay, but a few hours later I'm wide awake. Sometimes it takes me hours to go back to sleep.

Lily felt fairly casual about the physical changes she noticed. She shared that her mother entered menopause with ease, perhaps because of her Japanese heritage. Historically, Japanese women have not experienced menopausal symptoms, presumably because of diets high in soy and low in meat consumption. According to her mother, none of the women on her side of the family experienced any difficulty phasing through this normal transition of a woman's life. But Lily's work demanded sharp, alert, and focused attention, which waned for her due to lack of sleep.

She began using a 10 percent progesterone cream every twelve hours for twenty-one days each month. This seemed to help with the insomnia, but because Lily felt sleepy during the day, she chose to apply it only at bedtime. Five months later, Lily told me that the sleep disturbances had returned, she had not bled for three months, and she now experienced vaginal dryness. Lily also complained of an increase in anxiety, the occasional heart palpitation, and forgetfulness.

Using a cream became less convenient, so I changed her formula to an oral capsule containing 1 mg of estradiol, 4 mg of estriol, and 100 mg of progesterone, which she took every twelve hours. The new symptoms reflected a decline in her estrogen as well as her progesterone levels. Lily took this for two months, at which point her period restarted on a regular basis. After eleven months, she felt so great that she discontinued the formula, thinking she no longer needed the hormonal support.

However, when Lily began to suffer from dry eyes, dry skin with outbreaks of eczema, dry vagina, an overnight thinning of her pubic hair, and the return of her disturbed sleep, she agreed to take the salivary hormonal analysis. This test evaluates hormone levels from a cellular perspective. Her DHEA levels pooled together registered at a borderline low of 3—the normal range is between 3 and 10. Lily's testosterone, estrone, estradiol, and estriol were all well within the normal range, considered to be the physiologic target. Her progesterone had practically bottomed out.

Previously, she did not experience signs of estrogen decline for very long, because her formula of a biestrogen with progesterone had stimulated her own estrogens back into production. But she had consistently maintained low progesterone for an extended period. Lily's new prescription, a combination of 100 mg of progesterone with 10 mg of DHEA, restored her sense of balance and alleviated her symptoms. At the time of this writing she has been on this formula for two years.

FEEL LIKE YOU'RE BLEEDING ALL THE TIME?

Beth's story, age forty-four

> *Not only am I bleeding every sixteen days, but my periods have be-*
> *come painful. This has been going on for several months. I never had*
> *cramps before. My breasts swell and become painful a couple of days*
> *before I start. I sleep well and don't have any hot flashes, night*
> *sweats, or any of the other things I've heard women experience in*
> *menopause, except one thing: I'm having pain with penetration. It*
> *feels like my yoni will rip open just as my husband begins to enter*
> *me. My libido seems fine, though perhaps a bit less over the past year.*
> *Am I in menopause?*

Beth, who was forty-four, had begun the perimenopausal process,
probably during the previous year. Her first prescription consisted of a
10 percent progesterone cream, one-quarter of a teaspoon beginning on
day seven of her cycle, which she applied to her skin. She began massaging vitamin E oil into the opening of her vagina, her introitus, on a daily
basis with the additional application of a low dose of vaginal estriol
cream at bedtime for two to three nights each week. Her next cycle
started on day twenty-five. Within that first month, her vaginal dryness
disappeared, as did the painful intercourse, and she discontinued the
vaginal estriol. She continued, however, to take her progesterone.

Six months later, her painless menses had become more spotting than
an actual flow. Intercourse began to hurt again. She resumed the vaginal
estriol for one week and began taking sublingual drops of 1.25 mg of
biestrogen in addition to the progesterone. Beth returned in six months
to report that she had doubled her estrogen drops and noticed she felt
better. Her new formula became 2.5 mg of biestrogen with 100 mg of
progesterone twice a day, until suddenly her libido bottomed out. She
also wanted to simplify her regime, so her combination formula changed
from a cream to oral capsules. Beth was not ready to relinquish her sex
life and wanted an immediate remedy. Applying testosterone cream directly to her clitoral area not only restored her libido but she described
her vagina as feeling healthy, alive, and pain-free again.

The next change for Beth occurred eight months later with a slight increase in the biestrogen to 3.5 mg, which served her for about five months when her menses became irregular. She spotted one month, skipped the next, and began to bleed every two weeks. Beth's joints became achy as well. I increased her biestrogen to 5 mg and added a remedy specific for the health of her joints; she also made some dietary adjustments. She took homeopathic Rhus Tox 200C four times a day, began taking glucosamine, increased her calcium to 1,200 mg with 600 mg of magnesium, and added 30 mg of both boron and zinc. Her biggest challenge was eliminating sugar and decreasing her carbohydrates.

> *I love sweets, my entire family does. I guess we have an addiction to sugar, and to pasta, and to breads, pastries, all the gooey stuff that tastes so good but is so bad. I'll try this, but I do not think it will be easy.*

A year and a half later, she admitted to making none of the dietary changes and noticed more arthritis-like symptoms. Although she experienced some relief with the remedies, she had concerns of it progressively worsening. She had also developed some digestive disturbances. We talked about how eliminating sugar might actually eliminate her joint pain and her sudden flatulence. Six months later, she declared:

> *I've cut out dairy, definitely downscaled the sugar, and I hardly eat pasta or bread now. My energy has been lower since I've made these changes, though in general I feel pretty good.*

I added 5 mg of DHEA to her combination formula, which helped with the low energy level she had developed since she eliminated much of her sugar sources. Her cycles dwindled to regular periods of spotting for three or four days each month at the time she expected her menses. During the five years we worked together, Beth's hormones shifted and her formulas needed continual adjustment from her initial prescription. She continues to take this most recent prescription. Beth checked in with me on a regular basis, every three to six months, and kept me informed of changes as she noticed them, the positive as well as the negative. This gave me the information I needed to fine-tune her hormone formula and readjust her hormonal balance.

Beatrice's experience, age forty-four

I'm bleeding every two weeks, though no cramps, thank God. Lately I've been waking up at night drenched in sweat, and then I get these deep chills. My husband says I've become quite moody, though I didn't notice. However, I have been feeling irritable and maybe a bit more anxious than usual. Before my periods became all screwy, and I could know when I ovulated, I noticed my energy seemed to go down just after ovulation.

Beatrice chose to evaluate her hormones with a blood test, because her insurance would pay for it, and not the salivary analysis. We discovered that her progesterone was significantly low for where she was in her cycle. She began taking 100 mg of progesterone twice a day, which was actually not enough to completely resolve the night sweats and sleep disturbances. Although her next menses arrived on day twenty instead of day twelve or fourteen, we doubled her bedtime dosage of progesterone to 200 mg. Two and a half months later, the night sweats had decreased to only one or two nights before her menses would start. Because her progesterone continued to measure low, she began taking a double dose in the morning also.

Her next blood test revealed an extremely low testosterone level of 3, and with this particular lab the normal range is 22 to 80. Needless to say, Beatrice needed testosterone, 3 mg of which was added to each of her progesterone capsules, with additional plain progesterone that she could take at night if she needed it. Her menses now occurred every twenty-five days and continued to do so for seven months. Her next test results showed her testosterone had increased to 38, her progesterone had improved but remained in the lower ranges of normal, and her DHEA measured as low normal.

Over the next six months she felt significantly better, with more consistent energy, as well as continued regularity of twenty-seven to twenty-eight days in her cycle while taking a daily combination dosage of 200 mg of progesterone, 10 mg of DHEA, and 8 mg of testosterone, with additional progesterone at bedtime. Finally, her own progesterone production kicked into gear and her dosage needed to be decreased. The primary signal for this change occurred when Beatrice began to feel drowsy in the morning after she took her progesterone. Her hormonal analysis confirmed that her progesterone, testosterone, and DHEA levels had risen. I tried graduating her progesterone, beginning with 35 mg on days two through ten, 50 mg on days eleven through twenty-three, and 75 mg on days twenty-four through twenty-eight, twice a day. Her cycle became closer together within the first month, occurring on day nineteen, then the next cycle on day eleven, and the following one on day sixteen.

Taking 75 mg of progesterone twice a day over the next three months stabilized her cycle into the every twenty-five- to twenty-eight-day pattern. But Beatrice began feeling more aggressive and irritable, having more PMS. She is now forty-six years old and experiencing her first set of hot flashes, even though her estrogens have always measured within the normal range. Rather than giving her estrogen right away, I increased her progesterone back up to 100 mg along with 5 mg of DHEA per dose, which worked well for the next seven months. At that time, her stress levels had risen appreciably with more than one family crisis and a divorce.

Even with all the increase of stress, Beatrice's cycles were averaging about every twenty-five days. But the hot flashes returned, though not the sweating, along with breast tenderness and headaches before her menses. Keeping her progesterone and DHEA dosages consistent, I added 2.5 mg of biestrogen into her total daily dose. Over the next eight months, her prescription continued to be adjusted by increasing and decreasing either her estrogen or her progesterone. During this time, she experienced three twenty-eight-day cycles, one twenty-day cycle, and the other four ranged from twenty-three to twenty-five days apart. As her stress levels continued to climb, so did her adrenal exhaustion, which necessitated adrenal support, as well as separating each hormone so she could adjust her dosage on a daily basis, depending upon what was happening in her everyday life and her stress levels.

Since Beatrice is not yet postmenopausal, and may indeed have many years to go, her hormones and formulas required to support hormonal balance will continue to require adjustments and change over time. Not every woman goes through as many changes as Beatrice has to date. But I wanted you to see how working with hormonal supplementation is an ongoing communication between a woman and her prescribing practitioner. Beatrice's commitment to take only natural hormones and her desire to work with her body's signals, to optimize her health and her sense of well-being, began with clear choices, and a tenacity that persists.

FLOODING

It can be either a bit frightening or completely terrifying to experience a profuse gushing of blood pouring out of you, hour after hour. Some women actually think they might hemorrhage to death. Flooding that becomes unstoppable despite hormonal and other supplemental treatments may elicit the need for a D&C (dilation and curettage, or suction curettage), a surgical procedure during which the cervix is dilated to accommodate the insertion of surgical instruments through the vagina to essentially clean out the inside of the uterus. A D&C removes clots, pooled blood, and tissue fragments from the uterus, and provides samples of endometrium for pathological examination. There have been such severe instances of hemorrhaging during the menopausal process that women have been given hysterectomies.

Flooding, or metrorrhagia, occurs when the endometrium buildup becomes too thick, and the uterus does not effectively shed it on its own. Flooding usually results from sustained low progesterone levels and responds well to compounded phytogenic natural progesterone. This is covered more in Chapter 11's discussion of uterine fibroids, with which it is commonly associated.

Felipa's experience, age forty-eight

I've been bleeding continuously for twenty-three days and it's wearing me down. It is not gushing every day. But some days I literally must sit on the toilet for what feels like hours. It's become difficult to leave the house or be very far away from the toilet. I'm starting to feel woozy or dizzy and I cannot concentrate very well. The other day I almost fainted, but I caught myself just in time. And my poor husband, he doesn't know what to do with me. I never want to make love anymore. Who would want to with all this blood?

Felipa's cycles had been regular for most of her life except in adolescence when she first began menstruating. In fact, over the previous five years, her flow became quite light. Felipa did not have uterine fibroids or any other pelvic pathology. My primary concern was to stop the bleeding, treat the anemia that resulted from her excessive blood and iron loss, and build up her strength and stamina.

Initially she took 100 mg of progesterone every four hours along with homeopathic Sabina 1M every twelve hours, for three doses. Felipa needed the nutritional support of iron, high protein, iron-rich foods, and an increase in fluids to replenish her losses. Nourishment with Chinese herbs was called for, so she began taking Sea of Qi Formula to assist with the prolonged bleeding, dizziness, and generalized weakness, and Bupleurum and Tang Kuei Formula to address the excessive bleeding. Both formulas worked with her fatigue. Exhausted, Felipa, who was so accustomed to taking care of everyone else, needed permission to take naps to help her get more rest.

The bleeding trickled down to light mucousy spotting within twenty-four hours and stopped in two days. The high dosage of progesterone changed to 100 mg twice a day, with extra on hand in case the bleeding restarted prematurely. This held her for the next twenty-one days, when her menses began, albeit a week early. She expressed fears and concerns about flooding again, which were quickly set to rest by a normal flow. Her libido returned with resolution of the flooding. The Chinese herbal formula was discontinued after two months.

Felipa experienced episodes of flooding twice more over the next year, each time remedied with progesterone. When the episodes occurred, Felipa faced her fears of losing herself in pools of blood. The fears resolved with the increase of progesterone and the addition of Aconite 200C every four hours on the day she felt utterly convinced that she would bleed to death. The bleeding slowed to a normal flow and she did not die.

Over the next two years her cycles began to fade away until she became postmenopausal and needed estrogen support. Felipa felt so relieved when her cycles disappeared that at first she did not want to take any estrogen for fear of restarting her menses, but the hot flashes and dry skin got to her. A low dose of 1.25 mg of biestrogen with 100 mg of progesterone continues to serve her well.

SIMPLY UNPREDICTABLE AND IRREGULAR

Ivanna's story, age forty-seven

> My periods have always been predictable, every twenty-seven days.
> It's been three months, and other than feeling as if it's on the verge of
> happening any day, there's no sign. And now I guess I might be hav-
> ing hot flashes, though I'm not exactly sure what they are. I just seem
> to feel hot much of the time.

Ivanna's hormone analysis showed that she was low in everything except
testosterone, which was at a normal level. At forty-seven, with her first
symptom of irregular menses and feelings of excess heat, she entered
perimenopause. Her first formula was 5 mg of biestrogen with 100 mg
of progesterone and 5 mg of DHEA. Because she felt very unfocused and
grieved the loss of her former self, I gave her homeopathic Ignatia 1M,
to take at twelve-hour intervals for three doses, and daily exercises to
help her feel more grounded and connected to the earth. Initially, Ivanna
felt better. When she returned to see me four months later, she confessed
that she took her prescription inconsistently once the hot flashes vanished.

> Now I feel kinda edgy. I seem to have all this nervous energy and I'm
> not sleeping well. I did get a period a month and a half ago. Maybe I
> could get more in the habit of taking something in a pill form instead
> of the cream. The cream felt nice, when I remembered to use it.

These changes were easy to make. Her next combination was in an oral
capsule with the same amount of progesterone and DHEA, but I lowered her biestrogen to 3.5 mg, and asked her to follow up with me in
three weeks instead of three months.

She did not do well with the oral approach. Ivanna actually felt
worse, with increasing symptoms of PMS daily and her digestive disturbances becoming flatulently apparent. It seemed she did not absorb the
hormones well through the gut. We talked about different ways to use
the cream more consistently.

I suggested she place the pot of cream in an easily accessible and visi-

ble place for the morning dose—for example, next to her toothbrush.
After applying the morning dose, she should place it on her pillow. That
way if she didn't immediately remember her bedtime dose, she would
when she had to move it to get into bed. I then suggested that if she had
difficulty remembering to rotate the application spots on her body each
day, she begin the week with an upper-body location and work her
way downward as the week progressed. Ivanna also experimented with
her dose and discovered that she felt her best when she took one and a
half doses at bedtime and half a dose in the morning. Her menses became more of a light spotting for two days a month with more predictable patterns, her energy improved, and she began sleeping better.

AUGMENTING NATURAL TREATMENTS

Homeopathy
- *Aconite* stops uterine hemorrhage that is commonly accompanied by
  the enormous fear of impending death.
- *Belladonna* stops sudden onset uterine hemorrhage, especially when
  the bleeding is bright red and feels hot.
- *Ferrum* helps the flushing that accompanies excessive bleeding.
- *Calcarea Carbonica* helps with metrorrhagia in menopause.
- *Ipecacuanha* helps with sudden onset, bright red gushing blood, with-
  out clots, along with nausea, vomiting, and fainting.
- *Kali Ferrocyanatum* helps profuse, painless hemorrhaging that results
  in radical anemia (uterine fibroids).
- *China Officinalis* helps with floods with dark blood.
- *Crocus Sativus* is helpful in enduring uterine hemorrhage with dark,
  stringy clots.
- *Sabina,* a primary remedy for uterine problems, helps to stop hemorrhages accompanied by intense pain, active gushing, and often with
  clots and a bright red flow.

Herbal Helpers for Menstrual Irregularities

For Flooding and Hemorrhaging
- *Cinnamon:* 20 drops twice a day to help regulate cycle, 10 drops every
  fifteen to twenty minutes to slow flooding

- *Lady's Mantle:* 10 drops three times a day for one to two weeks before menses to help control hemorrhaging and prevent flooding. It may cause contractions of the uterus.
- *Shepherd's Purse:* 20 drops four times a day to decrease heavy bleeding and 15 to 20 drops held under the tongue four to six times a day for flooding.

For Irregular Bleeding
- *Bupleurum and Tang Kuei Formula*
- *Dong Quai:* 20 drops of the tincture four times a day for one week to initiate a late or absent menses, but prolonged usage of dong quai alone can result in heavy bleeding.
- *Gingerroot tea*
- *Nettle leaf tea:* one cup a day
- *Sea of Qi Formula*
- *Vitex:* 20 drops three times a day
- *Wild yam:* 20 drops three to four times a day for midcycle spotting
- *Witch hazel:* 20 drops four times a day

SEX, LIBIDO, AND ORGASM . . .

It is very common for women whose hormones are not in balance to lose interest in sex. Sometimes, this has emotional roots, but often the pragmatic issue of pain from vaginal dryness dispels desire. If hormone levels are too low, there is simply no libido at all. Pain plus lack of desire equals zero pleasure.

Hormonal deficiencies, though, are not the only cause for a woman's libido to disappear. Thyroid dysfunction and adrenal exhaustion also play a significant role in the loss of healthy sexual function, as are a poorly nourished body, mind, or soul. With the many changes that occur physically and emotionally during the menopausal process, it is no wonder the libido evaporates for many women. If a woman feels that her life is out of control, if she is gaining weight, exhausted, and on an emotional roller coaster, her sensual self becomes nonexistent. She looks into the mirror and barely recognizes herself.

Balancing hormones to address any of the possible accompanying symptoms is crucial in the process of reestablishing a healthy libido, even if you're not sexually active. Our sexual energy and creativity are intertwined. Healthy sexual energy supports our creative self. Many menopausal symptoms interfere with sexual function, being orgasmic, or simply having an interest in sex at all. These include:

1. Unpredictable menses, especially if your periods have gotten closer together. Bleeding every other week with a heavy flow results in a lack of sexual energy simply because sex can be uncomfortable.
2. Migraines knock a woman out of all normal functioning and usually negate any sexual desire. Movement worsens the migraine, as does elevation of blood pressure, both of which normally occur during lovemaking.
3. Mental or physical fatigue and exhaustion, whether from insomnia, sleep disturbances, or any other potential cause, leave no energy for sex. If you are too tired to do the important tasks of daily life, then sex will be the last thing on your mind.
4. Night sweats make you feel hot, sweaty, sticky, and perhaps more odiferous than ever before in your life. And then your partner declares: "Come on, girl, I wanna make you sweat." Oh please, you think, not on your life.
5. Pain anywhere—joints, muscles, tendons, bones, uterus, breast, teeth, gums, bladder, vagina, take your pick—distracts you to the point that there is no way you can feel sexy. Intercourse aggravates vaginal, bladder, uterine, or ovarian pain, which should be treated before attempts to resume normal sexual activity.
6. Digestive disturbances . . . now honestly, who feels sexy when their belly is swollen with the bloat, they're having gas pains, or farting?
7. Bodily changes such as weight gain, particularly from the waist down; loss of breast tissue; skin drying up, tearing, or breaking out with acne; loss of grace in movements; hair anywhere it never used to be; and loss of muscle tone all alter one's perception of self. We do not open our body sexually when we feel shut down and not beautiful.
8. Any of the twenty-five psychological and emotional symptoms of perimenopause or menopause (pages 143–145) may negate or certainly impede sexual desire and its meaning in one's life.

DISCOVER THE PATTERN TO YOUR CYCLES

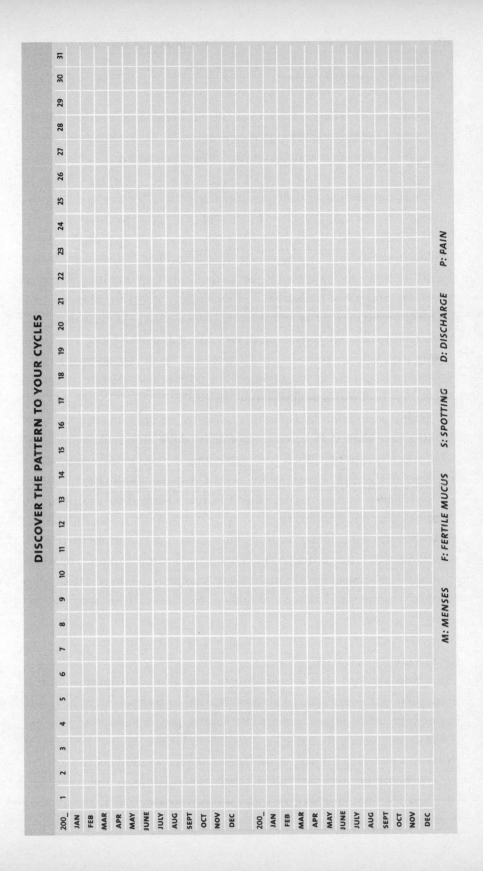

M: MENSES   F: FERTILE MUCUS   S: SPOTTING   D: DISCHARGE   P: PAIN

Sabina's story, age forty-nine

> *My biggest complaint is sex, or the lack of it and no longer caring. This*
> *does not feel normal to me. It's not my husband's fault, though, it's my*
> *vagina's. Everything was fine on my last annual exam and Pap smear*
> *according to my doctor. But she didn't offer me anything for my*
> *vagina, which feels so tight and bone-dry most of the time. I used to*
> *enjoy sex, but now it hurts and I am simply not interested anymore.*

Sabina described her cycles, which were becoming closer together and
lighter in flow. She experienced occasional night sweats that disturbed
her sleep, and a hot flash now and then. Her estrogens, progesterone,
and testosterone levels were low, which was no surprise. In a combination oral capsule, she took 6 mg of biestrogen and 100 mg of progesterone twice a day. In response to her testosterone deficiency and lack of
libido, she began gently massaging half a gram of testosterone cream, 10
mg per gram, directly on her clitoral area twice a day.

Sabina needed the testosterone treatment for only one month. During that time she rediscovered her sex drive and became easily orgasmic.
The oral formula nourished her fragile vaginal tissue and repaired the
integrity of the skin, reestablishing normal vaginal secretions.

Two and a half years later, her formula changed to less estrogen,
decreasing to 4 mg, with progesterone remaining the same, and 2.5 mg
of DHEA was added. Her healthy libido continues to sustain itself without additional testosterone. Although during the time Sabina's stress levels increased tremendously due to an unexpected family crisis, with
adrenal support and vitamin and mineral supplementation she managed
to hold her own.

Laia's experience, age sixty-three

Laia, a lovely sixty-three-year-old woman in a loving relationship, had
been unable to transcend the despair induced by painful intercourse and
an inability to be orgasmic since she became menopausal. She also suffered from frequent bladder infections. Every time she and her partner
tried to express their love physically, her vagina would tear, causing her
to experience terrible pain and bleeding. When she first came to see me,
she had been taking Prempro without receiving any relief. She cried as
she spoke.

I just can't go on like this anymore. I love my husband and, quite frankly, I used to love sex. The last doctor added vaginal Premarin to fix this nuisance, but it didn't do anything except make me feel all gooey inside.

Her first formula included 5 mg of triestrogen with 100 mg of progesterone and 5 mg of testosterone in a transdermal cream designed as a twice-daily application. Six weeks later, she returned after extensive travels. Laia blushed and giggled as she spoke of their sojourn:

I really pushed myself rather intensely. We hiked until I exhausted myself. But my spirits have been so uplifted since I started this prescription that I didn't care about feeling tired. And we made love and we made love. I'm talking about doing it twice a night. It was glorious! Before, we'd try to make love about once every four months— that was my recovery time—four months! Now, no pain, no bleeding, and, oh honey, it was delicious.

We experimented with two other formulas, increasing the estradiol and deleting the estrone, changing from a transdermal approach to taking it orally. But the original prescription has served her the best for the past three years. Laia applies one of her twice-daily doses to her skin, and the other she takes in an oral capsule.

OTHER NATURAL SUPPORT

Homeopathic Remedies
- *Aurum* for when sex drive is altered by grief or thoughts of suicide
- *Caladium* for when the sex drive is initially high and drops, followed by sexual inability
- *Causticum* for aversion to coition, often with vaginal/bladder burning
- *Conium* for marked sexual dysfunction
- *Graphites* for aversion to sex
- *Natrum Muriaticum* for when an aversion to sex develops, and for when painful intercourse occurs as a result of vaginal dryness
- *Onosmodium* for when there is a preoccupation with sex but a loss of libido
- *Sepia* for when a woman experiences aggravation from her hormonal

imbalance and from coition, often developing an aversion to being touched and to sex

Herbal Helpers
- *Damiana:* 375 mg up to three times a day
- *St. John's Wort:* 25 drops three times a day
- *Fenugreek tea:* drink daily for sweet-smelling sweat
- *Ginseng/Dong Quai*
- *Cinnamon* plus *Dragon Bone* and *Oyster Formula*

Nutritionals
Growth Hormone Release Extract (GHRE) comes in a sublingual spray and should be taken on an empty stomach, otherwise nausea occurs. GHRE enhances sensual sensations and stimulates vaginal fullness. The number of squirts per dose varies per person, though it is wise to start with twelve. Too many squirts can induce vomiting or uncontrollable deep sleep for three hours. If mixed with alcohol it causes central nervous system (CNS) depression. It should be used with caution and according to recommended doses only.

Natural Vaginal Lubricants
Massage the oil, cream, or ointment into the skin at the entrance of your vagina, the introitus, and inside your vagina as often as you feel the need (daily is okay). The following can be used to help during lovemaking. *Emerita,* made by Transitions for Health, Inc., is a formula designed to be used to assist in sustaining vaginal lubrication during extended lovemaking sessions.

- Almond or other vegetable oil
- Calendula cream
- Cocoa butter
- Coconut oil
- Comfrey ointment
- Plantain oil or ointment, especially if you have itching
- Vitamin E oil
- Emerita (contains some lovely ingredients—calendula, chamomile, ginseng, black walnut leaf—and is nurturing to sensitive vaginal tissue)

- *Avoid:* bubble baths, douches, soaps, panties with synthetic crotches, and panty hose, as these items promote vaginal dryness and the lack of adequate aeration. Thigh-highs or stockings requiring a garter allow a normal air flow through panties with breathable crotches and are far sexier than panty hose.

EXERCISE—NOURISH YOUR VAGINAL MUSCLES AND TISSUE

Wise words were spoken to me long ago by one of my teachers at the University of California at San Francisco. I will always remember her simple phrase in reference to the vagina: "If you don't use it, you lose it." And she was right. Sexual activity, *using it,* prevents vaginal atrophy and a decrease in vaginal lubrication. Sexual excitement infuses the pelvis and specifically the vaginal tissue with energy as well as expanding the cells. This expansion draws hydration directly into the membranes, literally plumping up vaginal and bladder cellular structures.

Women who don't "use it"— those who remain celibate even from self-love—"lose it" as they develop thinner bladder and vaginal tissue early in their hormonal decline transiting into menopause. This thinning is responsible for pain, lesions, infections, and the general lessening of desire.

Many women lose sight of the magical mysteries held within their vaginas. Reawaken this magic for yourself, even if you do not currently have a partner.

- *Sacred spot massage,* also known as the *G-spot* (named after the early sexologist Ernest Grafenberg), is a bulge that can be felt through the anterior vaginal wall. This area's blood vessels become engorged during sexual arousal and stimulation. When initially massaged, a woman may experience a sensation mimicking the urge to urinate. If sustained, this sensation transforms into sexual excitement, and over an extended period may bring orgasm to a higher stage, culminating in female ejaculation.

  Sacred spot massage brings your conscious awareness into your inner sanctum as well as giving you the opportunity to expand and contract your vaginal muscles, pumping energy and lubrication into your vagina, bringing deeper sexual pleasure. You can find this and other exercises that you can practice alone or with a partner in the book *Healing Love Through the Tao: Cultivating Female Sexual Energy,* by Mantak and Maneewan Chia.

• *Kegel exercises,* developed by Dr. Arnold Kegel, work the pelvic floor muscle (*pubococcygeus*), often referred to as the PC muscle, and increase awareness, strength, and circulation in your vaginal area as well as your sexuality. Identify the PC muscle by sitting on the toilet, with your legs relaxed and apart. Now start the flow of urine, and squeeze your vaginal muscles, without moving your legs, to the point that urination stops, then release your grip. You have just identified the muscles you want to exercise. However, do not practice this while urinating because it may cause urine to back up in the bladder and cause an infection. Actually, you can practice Kegels almost anytime, anywhere—while driving your car, chatting to a friend on the phone, or whenever you're just sitting still for a few moments—though this could get a bit tricky if you take it to the level of sexual arousal.

The action of contracting and releasing your vaginal muscles, repeatedly, strengthens and tones the vaginal walls, better supports your bladder, and enhances lubrication. Fill your bath and add your favorite essential oil scent, surround yourself with lit candles and nice music. As you are warmed and soothed by the water, "breathe" in through your vagina, contract your pelvic floor muscles and draw the muscles upward and deeper inward, allowing the water to enter. "Exhale" through your vagina, releasing the water back out into the tub. You will find this a more sensual way to practice Kegels. Let yourself feel sexually turned on if this happens naturally for you, but do not force it. Your vaginal integrity and tone will still benefit.

You can practice these exercises at different paces, alternating at your own comfortable tempo, and often. You may want to begin doing a series of ten "squeezes" five times throughout the day. Post a note that says "Squeeze" or "Pulse" or "Tighten" on your fridge, your mirror, or anywhere you pass to remind you.

1. Tighten your PC muscle, hold, and count to three. Relax.
2. Squeeze and relax your PC muscle in rapid succession, as quickly as you can.
3. Pull up your entire pelvic floor, then bear down as though you are pushing something out of you.

Another way to tone is by contracting the vaginal entry muscles around your finger(s), dildo, crystal egg, or other creative vaginal insert. Feel each of the higher layers of muscles as you continue to contract around the inserted item completely. Focus your breathing while you contract and release your muscles in a pulsing motion.

- *Toe-Tapping* is an exercise that calms the restless mind and body and opens the pelvic energy. (See page 181 for a detailed discussion.)

THE BURNING ZONE: CONDITIONS OF THE VAGINA, BLADDER, ANUS

The vagina, the bladder, the anus—how close together they can be . . . and how fragile the tissue becomes as hormonal nutrients disappear. When hormonal deficiency results in recurrent infections, adequate hormonal coverage is needed to eliminate the inflammatory process and restore integrity to these delicate tissues. Nourished skin no longer tears and decreases susceptibility to infections.

THE VAGINA/YONI, THE VULVA

As you have seen in the previous section, hormonal deprivation creates havoc with one's sex life. Beyond the sexual repercussions, vaginal changes and infections can be treated and often prevented by nourishing the vaginal tissue with adequate lubrication and compounded phytogenic hormones. Unless you are treating an active infection with a short-term douche, *do not* douche. Douching strips away the normal vaginal flora—the good bacteria—that keeps the vagina healthy and can increase vaginal dryness and irritation. To assist you in identifying infection, keep on hand a roll of Nitrazine or pH paper that ranges from 4.5 to 7.5.

Vaginal Dryness

Many women respond to their primary compounded phytogenic hormone formula and do not need any additional vaginal treatment. Others need a more direct approach. In addition to initiating systemic hormone therapy, you may need short-term vaginal therapy in the form of vaginal progesterone suppositories or estriol vaginal cream, typically applied every night for one to two weeks and two to three times a week over the following month. Vaginal progesterone suppositories are made in a variety of dosages ranging from 100 mg to 600 mg. Estriol vaginal cream, 2 mg per gram of cream, utilizes a smaller quantity of cream to accomplish the same nourishing action as a full applicator of a lower dose. A vagina full of cream may feel like a relief or it may feel quite goopy, especially if it continually squishes out. The goal is to coat the mucous membranes lining the vagina and infuse the hormonal nutrients directly into the tissue.

If you use an over-the-counter, nonprescription, natural progesterone or estrogen cream vaginally, make sure it does not contain alcohol. Alcohol burns fragile tissue and may increase dryness. Once your hormones find their balance, the vaginal treatment will no longer be necessary.

Nonhormonal Natural Treatments
1. Homeopathic Remedies

   • *Bryonia, Belladonna*, and *Lycopodium* for dryness
   • *Belladonna* and *Cantharis* for a hot, burning feeling
   • *Natrum Muriaticum* for intense pain with dryness
   • *Sulfur* for intense itching

2. Plain yogurt cools hot burning sensations when applied directly.
3. Comfrey cream, applied directly to affected area
4. Plantain ointment, applied directly, helps with itching and tissue repair.
5. Dong Quai taken orally stimulates increased lubrication.
6. Acupuncture stimulates the pelvic region.

See the previous section for other natural approaches to tonify and enhance vaginal lubrication.

Fragile labia and vulva, caused by hormonal deprivation, respond well to topical natural hormone creams, and sometimes better to compounded phytogenic testosterone cream than to estriol or progesterone. Apply a cream of 10 mg testosterone per gram two to four times a day for two to four weeks. Simultaneously, address your overall hormonal balance with a formula specific to your deficiencies.

Because there are many causes for vaginal irritation, itching, and burning, it is important to identify and treat the causative organism if infection develops. Vaginal infections, even in the presence of copious discharge and drainage, promote vaginal dryness.

Atrophy, atrophic vaginitis/vulvitis: Insufficient hormone production creates the changes manifesting as skin pallor, causing the vulva and vagina to have a blanched, shiny, whitish appearance. With increased thinning and sensitivity, the vagina and vulva become receptive to abrasions, dryness, and cracking of the tissue. Atrophy itself is not an infectious condition but it supports the climate that allows infections to develop; it is remedied by the hormonal suggestions noted above. However, in the presence of atrophic conditions with infection (vaginitis), characterized by vaginal discharge, pain, itching, burning, and a pH of 5.5–7.0, treat the specific infecting organism before using hormone creams vaginally.

Vaginal Infections

Many infections are treatable and curable without prescription drugs.

Vaginal yeast infections increase in the presence of hormonal imbalances, systemic candidiasis, and all immunocompromised and acidic conditions. The primary symptoms, which range from mild to severe, present with itching of the vulva and/or vagina, and vaginal discharge with an acidic pH of 4.5, which may be watery to a thick cottage-cheese texture. It is possible to have a yeast infection with only vulvar itching and no internal vaginal symptoms, or with only urinary symptoms present.

Natural Treatments

1. Y-Stat vaginal suppositories (by Bezwecken Transdermal Systems, Inc., and sold only to practitioners) contain 50 mg of berberis, 50 mg of calendula, 100 mg of hydrastis root, and 600 mg of boric acid. Insert one suppository into the vagina at bedtime or at the first sign of a known yeast infection. One application may resolve the infection if caught at the earliest onset of development. In moderate cases, use three nights in a row; in severe cases, use twice a day for up to fourteen days.
2. Colloidal silver douche, 2 teaspoons in 1 cup of water, daily
3. Acidophilus in a capsule that has not previously been refrigerated and contains lactobacilli; follow instructions for Y-Stat, above.

4. Boric acid: Place pharmaceutical-grade boric acid in 600 mg capsules and use vaginally; follow instructions for Y-Stat, above.
5. Dietary support includes eliminating sugars, carbohydrates, and acidic foods.

Cervicitis, inflammation of the cervix, may be independent of other infections or accompany them. In menopause, hormonal balance helps prevent cervicitis, in the absence of STDs. Cervicitis alone has no noticeable odor to the white, creamy secretions with a pH that varies from 4.5 to 5.5.

Natural Treatments
1. Progesterone suppositories: 200–600 mg placed next to the cervix at bedtime, for seven to ten days.
2. Colloidal silver: 2 cc injected onto the cervix at bedtime for seven days. Get ready for bed first and finish toilet needs. Use a syringe *without the needle,* draw the colloidal silver up into the syringe, and lie on your back with a pillow or two under your hips to elevate your pelvis. Part your legs, insert the syringe into your vagina, and push the plunger, injecting the colloidal silver as high as you can. Tilt your pelvis back for a few moments. You may want to plug the opening of your vagina with half of an organic tampon to prevent leakage.
3. Folic acid: 10 mg a day for one to three months to increase the production of new, healthy cervical cells. If your Pap smear shows atypical cells or mild dysplasia (noncancerous cells), continue taking 10 mg of folic acid for up to six months and consider additional cervical treatment as needed per your practitioner's recommendation. Repeat Pap to assure cure.

Bacterial vaginosis (BV, previously known as Gardnerella), an infection caused by specific bacteria, is easily diagnosed by viewing a sample of vaginal secretions under a microscope. Vaginal symptoms include a creamy discharge with a fishy odor and a pH environment of 5.0–5.5. If your discharge has a fishy odor, pH of 5.0–5.5, and you are not at risk for having another infection or STD concurrently, try the following approaches.

Although BV is no longer considered an STD, if you develop it and you are sexually active, you share it with your partner. Men rarely become symptomatic but will harbor the bacteria in the base of their urethra, and return it to your vagina during ejaculation or in preejaculatory secretions, even if your man holds his seed. To help prevent BV, avoid rectal to vaginal contamination through personal hygiene after passing stool, and abstain from alternation between vaginal and anal intercourse during a continuous lovemaking session.

Natural Treatments

Douche twice a day for up to seven days with:

1. Colloidal silver: mix 2 teaspoons with 1 cup of water, or
2. Hydrogen peroxide: mix ¼ cup with 1 cup of warm water. If you also have a propensity for yeast add 2 tablespoons of acidophilus to the hydrogen peroxide and water, or
3. Betadine: mix 2 tablespoons with 1 cup of water, or
4. Herbal C or other herbal vaginal suppositories designed to treat bacteria: insert 1 suppository twice a day.

For *him,* for seven days:

1. Artestatin, a Chinese herbal formula: 3 tablets three times a day, or
2. Colloidal silver: 1 teaspoon three times a day, held under the tongue before swallowing

Note: If symptoms do not respond to the above, treat with prescription Metrogel or Flagyl.

Sexually active women, especially if you have more than one partner or are not mutually monogamous, need to remain mindful of sexually transmitted infections. STDs do not discriminate as to age, or how nice you might be. If vaginal dryness has become an issue, you'll want to use water-based lubricants, which do not cause condoms to dissolve.

If you have a common and treatable sexually transmitted infection, avoid sexual contact during times of infection.

Herpes simplex virus (HSV) is contracted through direct skin-to-skin contact in vaginal, anal, or oral sex if your partner has the virus actively circulating locally or systemically. The infected area is contagious from its prodromal (preliminary) stage, even if there are no visible signs, through the outbreak, and until the skin returns to normal. Hormonal balance decreases stress to the immune system and decreases the frequency of herpes outbreaks. There is no cure through Western medicine, only palliative treatment to suppress the activity of the virus into remission. However, I have seen long-term disappearance of HSV for at least ten years, or longer, with alternative therapies. Absolute cure with these treatments remains unproven to date.

Natural Treatments

1. Your specific homeopathic constitutional remedy
2. Olive Leaf extract: 1,000 mg every six hours
3. Olivirex: 2 capsules three times a day
4. Colloidal silver: 1 teaspoon four times a day orally; can also be applied to blisters
5. Lysine: 1,000 mg every two hours at the first sign
6. Low-acid diet
7. Ume concentrate: drink 1 pea-size amount dissolved in water four to six times a day to decrease acidity
8. Immune-supportive diet and lifestyle

Trichomoniasis, caused by parasitic protozoa, causes a curable vaginitis characterized by a frothy, malodorous, greenish-gray discharge, with a pH of 5.0–5.5, that varies in color and induces burning, itching, and irritation inside the vagina and vulva, along with urinary frequency, urgency, and pain. Usually sex becomes painful. The traditional treatment is Flagyl, 2 grams, taken orally.

Natural Treatments

1. Homeopathic trichomonas
2. Olivirex: 2 capsules three times a day
3. Olive Leaf extract: 1,000 mg every six hours
4. Colloidal silver: full-strength douche

Do not resume sexual activity without a condom until your vaginal secretions have been reexamined under a microscope and are clear of trichomonads.

Chlamydia, often responsible for infertility when left untreated, may present with odorous or odor-free vaginal discharge, burning on urination, lower abdominal pain, or no symptoms at all. Traditionally, chlamydia is treated with antibiotics, but I have seen this resolve with a homeopathic chlamydia. Follow-up cultures that assure cure are important even if you are no longer concerned with fertility.

Human papilloma virus (HPV) can cause genital warts or be invisible. It is estimated that 85 percent of the population, at least in the Western world, has HPV. It may appear on a Pap smear if it is cervical HPV. A woman with HPV can be symptom free or have vulvar itching, pain, and inflammation. A test you can do on yourself to see if you have vulvar HPV is to apply a 5 percent vinegar solution to your vulva. Wait three minutes and look at yourself with a strong light source, magnifying glass, and mirror. If HPV is present, you will see white opaque patches, acetowhite epithelium (AWE), on your skin and may experience burning. As with other viral infections, Western medicine does not provide a cure. However, as with HSV, I have witnessed not only long-term resolution of symptoms but normal test results.

Natural Treatments

1. PapilloDerm cream (made by Bezwecken and sold only to practitioners), applied twice daily
2. Colloidal silver, liquid or gel, applied twice daily
3. Immune-supportive diet and lifestyle

Other pathogens, potentially sexually shared, cause disease and warrant treatment and immune support. Viruses include hepatitis, cytomegalovirus (CMV), human immunodeficiency virus (HIV), Epstein-Barr virus (EBV), enteric viruses, and *Molluscum contagiosum.* Bacteria include *Neisseria gonorrhoea* (GC), mycoplasma, group B streptococcus, staphylococcus, syphilis, and various enteric bacteria and protozoa. Another protozoan causes pinworms. Other parasites include pubic lice and mites that cause scabies. Although these are not treated with natural hormones, a balanced hormonal system supports your immune system.

THE BLADDER

Cystitis, urinary tract infections (UTIs), *interstitial cystitis* (IC), *urethritis,* and symptoms that mimic sensations of bladder infection develop as hormonal nutrients decrease support to the bladder region. Vaginal infections without noticeable discharge may fool a woman into thinking she has a bladder infection. Burning and/or pain upon urination, the urge to urinate, and frequent urination are the most common symptoms.

Natural Treatments

1. *Compounded phytogenic hormones:* Balanced hormones help maintain the integrity of the tissue, repair thinning vaginal and bladder walls, and restore tone.
2. Drink 2 liters to 1 gallon of pure water throughout the day.
3. Void every two hours, or more often. Then drink another glass of water.
4. Acidify your urine with unsweetened cranberry juice—when you tire of drinking plain water or herbal teas, add some cranberry juice to your water.
5. Avoid alcoholic beverages, all forms of caffeine, citrus, and chilies—they irritate the bladder.
6. Urinate, cleanse, and rinse thoroughly with water after lovemaking to decrease the risk of developing a bladder infection. During lovemaking, normal bacteria are dislodged and can migrate into the bladder. Voiding flushes the bacteria from inside the urethra and cleansing your perineum keeps bacteria from gaining access to the urethral portal.
7. Homeopathic remedies:

   - *Aconite* for urine retention and is marked with fear
   - *Apis* for scalding pain on urination
   - *Belladonna* for hot and throbbing pain on urination
   - *Berberis* for cutting pains to the urethra and the meatus, pain and urges worsened by motion and urination
   - *Borax* for bladder pain with urinary retention
   - *Cantharis* for intense burning before, during, and after urination
   - *Capsicum* for chronic urethritis and for bladder and urethral pain that is worse after urination and with coughing

- *Causticum* for burning, frequent urges, and urinary retention
- *Hydrophobinum* for strong urges with UTI
- *Lycopodium* for painful urges
- *Medorrhinum* for recurring cystitis, nephritis
- *Natrum Carbonicum* for pain at the end of urination, urethral irritation with burning and stinging, and chronic cystitis
- *Nux Vomica* for the constant urge to urinate small amounts, and for painful retention
- *Pulsatilla* for cystitis and pyelonephritis (pelvic and kidney infections)
- *Sarsaparilla* for burning and frequent urges, and pain at the end of urination
- *Sepia* for frequency and sudden urgency
- *Staphysagria* for cystitis from intercourse, urethritis, frequent urges
- *Terebinthina* for terrible burning pain and urine that smells of violets

8. Western herbs

- *Corn silk tea:* To soothe the bladder, drink copious amounts, freely, throughout the day. Shuck ears of corn and separate the silken threads. Steep the threads in boiled water. Corn silk is also available in herbal capsules—handy if corn is out of season.
- *Black currant:* 15–20 drops three times a day helps prevent urinary infections while at the same time nourishing the adrenal glands.
- *Yarrow tea:* To help tonify the bladder as well as fight infection, drink once or twice a day.
- *Uva Ursi:* 10–20 drops three to six times a day for one to two days, then three times a day for up to ten days, for infection

9. Chinese herbs: Many formulas work to help tonify the bladder and kidneys, addressing symptoms of urinary pain, retention, infection, and excessive or nocturnal urination, or difficulty urinating.

Urinary incontinence is defined by the uncontrolled loss of urine. Commonly experienced in menopause, incontinence may result from weakened or injured pelvic floor muscles secondary to pregnancies, trauma, or surgeries; thinning of the bladder wall from lack of hormones; recurrent cystitis; the weight of uterine fibroids or ovarian cysts; chronic constipation and straining to pass stool; and alcohol abuse.

Stress incontinence is urine leakage caused by coughing, laughing, lifting, jumping, running, sneezing, vomiting, or any other activity that stresses the bladder.

Urge incontinence is the leakage of urine immediately with the urge to void.

Natural Treatment

1. Compounded phytogenic hormones that are formulated specifically to fit your needs
2. Pelvic floor exercises to strengthen bladder support
3. Meditation and biofeedback
4. Scheduled voiding—empty your bladder completely every sixty to ninety minutes, while awake, never allowing your bladder to become entirely filled or overfilled with urine. Over the next few days, begin expanding the periods between voiding, increasing over time to intervals of three to four hours, more if you tolerate it comfortably. Never let your bladder get too full as you lengthen these intervals. If incontinence returns, decrease the time to whatever works best for you.
5. Cranberry juice, without sugar
6. Avoid alcohol, caffeine, refined sugars, and tobacco.
7. Drink pure water and herbal teas throughout the day.
8. Avoid surgery.
9. Avoid drugs such as diuretics, antidepressants, sleeping pills, and tranquilizers.
10. Begin immediate treatment at the first signs of a UTI.
11. Homeopathic remedies (unless specified, these help with both stress and urge incontinence):

    - *Apis* for stress incontinence, especially from coughing
    - *Arsenicum Album*
    - *Cantharis* for incontinence or dribbling after urination
    - *Causticum*
    - *Hydrophobinum* for incontinence caused by the sound of running water
    - *Natrum Muriaticum* for stress incontinence and for "shy bladder," the inability to urinate in front of another

- *Pulsatilla*
- *Sepia*
- *Zincum*

12. Chinese herbal formulas such as Essential Yang, Nourish Essence, and Sea of Qi
13. Black cohosh—20 drops twice a day for two to four weeks

THE ANUS AND THE ANORECTAL CANAL

Hemorrhoids are a single or multiple mass of dilated veins in the anorectum that are located inside the canal or protrude externally. An *anal fissure* is an ulcerated line on the margin of the anus. As hormones decline, the fragility of the anal tissue can increase as it does in the bladder, vagina, vulva, and perineum. Hormonal balance helps maintain the integrity of anal tissue as well.

Natural Treatments
1. Compounded phytogenic hormones that are tailored specifically for your profile—balanced hormones help maintain the integrity of the tissue
2. Avoid constipation by

- Having an adequate fluid intake
- Drinking 1 cup of hot water first thing in the morning
- Eating blackstrap molasses—1–3 tablespoons—stirred into yogurt
- Eating a high-fiber diet
- Eating raw bran—1 tablespoon in 10 ounces of water one to three times a day
- Getting adequate regular exercise
- Responding to bowel urges; do not strain to pass stool
- Getting adequate, quality sleep

For hemorrhoids and fissures:

1. Topical cold compresses
2. Witch hazel packs

3. Homeopathic remedies are abundant; these are the most common.

- *Aloe* to treat hemorrhoids with marked congestion, bunched like grapes, and ones that are responsive to cold water
- *Belladonna* for rectal dryness, constipation, and hemorrhoids with exquisite pain and congestion
- *Bryonia* for constipation, passing dry and hard stool, and rectal dryness
- *Calcarea Phosphoria* for internal hemorrhoids that protrude with the passage of stool, possibly with diarrhea
- *Capsicum* if you also have colitis, heartburn, or significant thirst after passing stool
- *Collinsonia* for hemorrhoids and rectal fissures accompanied by a rectal sensation of fullness with small, sharp sticks; constipation and hard stool
- *Graphites* for fissures, and for constipation alternating with diarrhea
- *Hamamelis* for bleeding hemorrhoids
- *Ignatia* for rectal spasms, fissures, hemorrhoids, and prolapse; rectal sensation of a poker or knife inside
- *Kali Carbonicum* for painful, burning, itching hemorrhoids that are worse at night
- *Lachesis* for hemorrhoids that are congested and purplish
- *Natrum Muriaticum* for hemorrhoids that bleed, worse after hard stool
- *Nitricum Acidum* for great pain that lasts for hours after passing stool; anal fissures, fistula, abscess; rectal warts
- *Nux Vomica* for hemorrhoid pain that feels better with warmth and after passing of stool
- *Paeonia* for hemorrhoids, anal ulcerations, or rectal fissures with extreme pain after passing stool, pain so intense that it causes you to lie down holding your buttocks spread apart
- *Ratanhia* for hemorrhoids that protrude with the passage of stool, after which pain continues for hours; rectal sensation of burning or splintering
- *Sulfur* for hemorrhoids or fissures with rectal itching or burning; feels better with cold; offensive flatus and stool

4. Coat an external hemorrhoid with comfrey ointment and maneuver it into an internal position, if possible. Apply comfrey ointment to fissure two to four times a day.

5. Comfrey suppositories inserted after defecation

ARE YOU SLEEPING, *DORMEZ-VOUS, DORMEZ-VOUS?*

Are you feeling fatigued beyond belief, ready to collapse and watch the quality of your life rapidly deteriorate before your bleary eyes? Are you waking to drenched sheets saturated with your sweat, shivering as the ambient air whispers over your wet skin because you threw the covers off? Do nightmares echo from some dark corner of your psyche? Deep REM (rapid eye movement) sleep nourishes and heals us in ways transcending anything else. Without REM sleep, perceptions are distorted and the quality of life dissipates.

Sleeping pills sedate, and most addict you to their chemical components. Alcohol may knock you out initially, but it supports sleep disturbances a few hours later, leaving you awake, dehydrated, restless, and eventually with a headache and the inability to focus clearly. Both increase the stress on your liver, which is already working overtime with your hormones waning.

Shanti's story, age forty-eight

> I take naps now, every afternoon, along with Vitex and the Change of Life Formula. Nothing seems to help prevent those damned night sweats that keep me up half the night. I've been getting pretty irritable and I have all this nervous tension that I am clueless about. What have I got to be so anxious about? But if I don't start sleeping through the night, I feel like the little energy I have will disappear altogether. Oh, and I've completely lost my sex drive for five months now.

Shanti's sleep disturbances were caused by hot flashes that repeatedly awakened her in the night—night sweats. She had not yet tried anything hormonal, only herbs and vitamins. The first formula of 100 mg of progesterone included 5 mg of testosterone, to help work with her loss of libido and two small uterine fibroids, and 5 mg of DHEA to assist with her energy levels. According to her monthlong salivary analysis, her progesterone measured so low on days twenty-four through twenty-six that it was reported as zero. Her progesterone values never reached a level close to the normal range. The estrogens were within normal ranges, and her DHEA measured in the low normal limits.

Within two weeks, she felt much better. She was pleased about the return of her libido. Shanti began sleeping, undisturbed by night sweats, and she felt less fatigue, more energy. A year later, she began experiencing hot flashes, though only during the daytime. A low dose of 1.25 mg of biestrogen was added to her formula and she felt symptom-free for six months. Then suddenly the sleep disturbances returned. Her pelvic ultrasound showed shrinking fibroids, which was a delight because sometimes adding estrogen can cause uterine fibroids to grow.

Sometimes I'm having trouble falling asleep. I feel tired, but I just can't go to sleep. Instead, my mind is racing, wildly reminding me of all the things I should or should not do, and my legs just want to jiggle. Some nights I fall asleep easily but wake up around two-thirty or three in the morning.

Several issues needed to be addressed, all of which I felt contributed to Shanti's sleep disturbances. I wondered if the testosterone and DHEA might be a contributing factor, so I removed DHEA from her nighttime dose. As she no longer needed testosterone, that was deleted altogether. Her new prescription included the same amount of estrogen and progesterone with an increase of 10 mg of DHEA for her morning dose. At bedtime, she would take just the combination of biestrogen and progesterone, with the addition of 100 mg of progesterone for when she had difficulty falling asleep. Previously, Shanti had been taking only 500 mg of calcium, which is too low for a woman in the menopausal process. Her calcium was increased to 1,200 mg with 600 mg of magnesium, taken at bedtime. The increased calcium taken at bedtime not only enhanced the depth of her sleep, but resolved her restless legs.

According to Oriental medicine, around three in the morning is liver time. Liver function increases as hormones decrease. Additional liver support, therefore, in the form of herbal supplements, is sometimes necessary, though this was not true for Shanti. Yoga and tai chi enhanced her sense of balance. Two months later, she experienced a weeklong phase of sleeping poorly again. She tried a double dose of her combination formula only to awaken with a hangover. However, increasing her biestrogen has served her well ever since as did adding the bedtime active meditation of toe-tapping.

TOE-TAPPING

For restless legs and mind at night, try this simple active meditation.

Lie flat on your back with your legs out straight, comfortably close together. Relax your arms at your sides, palms facing upward.

Close your eyes.

Inhale calm, tranquil, soothing energy. Feel your heart slow its rhythm.

Exhale the day, the responsibilities, the distractions, the shoulds and should nots.

Continue to focus on your breathing and feel your breath through your lower belly. If you have never practiced abdominal breathing before, place your hands on your lower abdomen just below your navel. As you inhale, gently push your lower abdomen toward the sky. As you exhale, let your abdomen relax down toward the ground. This should not be done with tension in your muscles, but with a fluidity of movement guided by your breath.

Once you have established a peaceful rhythm, relax your arms out to your sides again at approximately a 45-degree angle, palms up.

Bring your feet together, heels gently touching. Move your big toes together, then let them fall outward and away from each other. Continue to bring your toes together and apart, together and apart, tapping them together as they touch. Continue to focus on your breathing while you tap your toes together at a pace that sets itself. The first time your toes touch, count one through ten in your mind; the second time, substitute the number twenty for ten; the third time thirty; and so on until you reach one hundred. Then restart with one to ten, to two hundred. Repeat this for as many times as you feel inclined. Five hundred is a good amount, but do less if you like.

This toe-tapping technique is not only very relaxing, but it also helps relax tension in the pelvis.

SUPPORTIVE NATURAL SUPPLEMENTS FOR SLEEP DISTURBANCES

Homeopathic Remedies

- *Nervoheel:* one tablet sublingually before bedtime soothes restlessness and nervous tension and helps with insomnia. Keep by your bed to take an extra dose when you awaken in the middle of the night.
- *Somcupin:* 20 drops three times a day and at bedtime deals directly with both the physical and psychic factors leading to insomnia and sleep disturbances.
- *Valerianaheel:* 10 drops three times a day and at bedtime relieves nervous anxiety, restlessness, nervous exhaustion, and insomnia.

Herbal Helpers

- *Hops:* 15 to 30 drops taken an hour before bedtime encourages a serene, more restful sleep.
- *Lavender essential oil,* dropped onto your pillow, or dried lavender flowers stuffed into a pillow pouch, will lull you into peaceful dreams, and will soothe your mind and body.
- *Nettle tea* nourishes the adrenals.
- *Sleep-Assure* (a combination formula of kavakava root, passionflower, valerian root, chamomile flower, gamma-aminobutyric acid [GABA], pyridoxal-5-phosphate, and melatonin): one tablet taken thirty minutes before bedtime to help relax and encourage a restful sleep

Nutritionals

- *Calcium:* 1,200–1,500 mg with 600–750 mg of magnesium (chewable, liquid, or capsules) taken at bedtime relaxes restless legs and minds while it calms the nervous system.
- *Melatonin:* One to three 1 mg sublingual tablets taken before bedtime helps with difficulties falling asleep. Dosages can go higher if needed and if directed by your practitioner. Some perimenopausal women experience disruption in their estrogen production while taking melatonin alone.

TOO HOT, TOO COLD, AH—JUST RIGHT

Perhaps you have seen a woman suddenly start to fan herself. Maybe her face turned bright red. *Hot flashes* vary from a mild increase in temperature, which for some women may even be a pleasant sensation, to an intense flush of heat with sweat dripping from the top of her head to the bottom of her feet. If a woman comes from a family unwilling to talk about "female troubles" or menopause—still surprisingly common—she may be told to "grin and bear it. It will go away, just ride it out." But this is totally unnecessary.

The hypothalamus is the part of your brain that contains neurosecretions, important for control of certain metabolic activities, such as maintenance of water balance, metabolism of sugar and fat, regulation of body temperature, and secretion by the endocrine glands. As estrogen levels drop, the hypothalamus becomes confused and thinks your body is overheating, and it responds to this decline of ovarian estrogen production by inducing the flush of heat experienced as a hot flash. It accomplishes this by releasing gonadotropin-releasing hormone in a pulsating manner, and this pulsation stimulates the release of lutenizing hormone (LH), which has a vasodilation effect (widening of blood vessels), causing the flush. This vasodilation allows you to release heat through your skin, and your sweat glands become activated to cool you down. Hot flashes come in bursts or waves due to this pulsating action, and can be primarily in the head and face, the upper body, or throughout the entire body. The patterns of hot flashes are often unpredictable and can occur at any time of the day or night, without warning, disturbing, distracting, or causing major disruptions for the woman experiencing them.

It is every woman's right to feel at her optimum, if possible. For the perimenopausal woman, the goal is not to return to feeling like nineteen again but rather to bring forward the wisdom of experiences to this transitional time and feel connected to our quintessential self.

Heidi's hot tale, age forty-six

Heidi, a high-powered executive, shared her first real hot flash experience.

> *Last week I had the hot flash from hell. Normally I don't wear face makeup, but for this presentation I was onstage and on camera. Just as I reached a crucial point in my project, it came. Like a wave from hell it swept over me from the top of my head to the tips of my toes, taking with it my makeup. I paused, looked down to discover my silk*

suit saturated with a layer of my face. Surrendering to the obvious, I interrupted my presentation with an old-lady joke. Help! I need damage control.

Heidi's first formula included 5 mg of biestrogen, 100 mg of progesterone, and 5 mg of testosterone. Her response was immediate and remarkable, and resolved all her symptoms. Other than removing the testosterone, Heidi has felt great on the same dose of estrogens and progesterone for the past four years.

Haleigh's experience, age forty-four

I am having hot flashes every hour on the hour, and all night long, too. I worked with herbs, but it didn't help. Not only do I not sleep because I flash and sweat all night long, but I have to get up to pee. Actually, I feel like I have to pee most of the time. My last menses was three months ago and my moods have bounced all over the place ever since. My skin has gotten very odd-looking, dry and thin. Oh, and I have no libido, zip, nada. I feel so exhausted and overwhelmed I don't know what to do.

Haleigh discontinued the hormonally related herbs and took 2.5 mg of triestrogen in sublingual drops and progesterone in a 10 percent cream twice a day. She also started drinking corn silk and yarrow tea to soothe and tonify her bladder. Because of her extended stress from the fatigue, I added 12.5 mg of DHEA to her progesterone cream. Within one week, she experienced no hot flashes, no mood swings, and was sleeping again.

Haleigh stayed on this regime for one year, during which her menses resumed a twenty-eight-day pattern, and her libido returned to normal. Then she began to experience hot flashes again, had three night sweats, increased irritability, and her libido bottomed out again, so she doubled her estrogen dose. Two months later, I added testosterone into the cream because her energy levels and libido did not respond to the increase in estrogen alone. She felt improvement within two weeks and continued on that combination for the next twelve months, when she wanted to switch to taking her combination in a capsule orally. For the next eleven months she took 5 mg of biestrogen, 100 mg of progesterone, and 7 mg of testosterone orally, twice a day.

Her cycles began to change again, becoming lighter and twenty-one days apart, and Haleigh noticed more headaches, verging on migraines. Her libido was much better and she had begun a yoga and workout program with weights. I lowered her biestrogen to 4 mg, the testosterone to 2 mg, with the 100 mg of progesterone, and added a separate 100 mg of progesterone for her to take at the first sign of a headache and every four hours until it abated. She preferred the progesterone in a cream to massage into her head with the migraines, feeling it to be more effective than the oral progesterone.

Haleigh's next formulary change was eight months later, to 5 mg of biestrogen with 100 mg of progesterone, when she needed an increase in estrogen for the return of hot flashes, night sweats, and awakening with brain fog. Her progesterone cream was increased to 200 mg per gram for her headaches. Because she had developed a slight increase in nipple hair and her low libido returned, the testosterone was taken out of her main systemic formula and put into a separate cream for her to massage into her clitoral region as needed. Now forty-nine, Haleigh finds that this approach continues to sustain her energy levels and resolve her hot flashes and other symptoms.

FOODS TO AVOID—THEY INCREASE HOT FLASHES

- Alcoholic beverages—even that glass of wine with dinner or the beer at the end of the day
- Caffeine of any variety—coffee, tea, soda, hot cocoa

A note on both coffee and alcohol: Not only do they increase heat, but they both dehydrate the cells and increase stress on the liver and kidneys.

- Hot beverages—they increase body heat
- Spicy foods—they stimulate and increase body heat
- Acidic foods
- Refined sugars
- Red meat
- Saturated fats

COOLING *FOODS TO ENJOY*

- Lots of pure water
- Mint herb tea and cooling herbs (refer to the next section on herbal helpers)
- Cucumber, jicama, celery—these also contain virtually no calories
- Yogurt, sugar- and all sugar substitute–free
- Whole grains, seaweeds
- Stevia—instead of sugar for sweetening
- Organic poultry, fresh fish
- Lots of fresh green leafy veggies
- Nuts and seeds, flaxseed
- Pomegranate seeds

AUGMENTING NATURAL SUPPORTS

Homeopathic Remedies

- *Aconite* for facial flushes and restlessness with fear and anxiety
- *Apis* for generalized hot flashes
- *Belladonna* for extreme changes in temperature and the sudden onset of hot flashes with skin turning bright red
- *Calcarea Fluorica* for hot flashes with heart palpitations, alternating with chills
- *Chamomilla* for hot flashes that are worse at night, causing restless sleep, weeping in sleep, and throwing the covers off
- *Ferrum* for profuse perspiration, and flashes that occur easily and are often accompanied by a red face
- *Gelsemium* for that sticky-all-over sweat with chills that alternate with hot flashes, and extreme fatigue
- *Kali Carbonicum* for flashes aggravated by heat and palpitations with hot flashes
- *Lachesis* for generally aggravated menopausal symptoms from the heat, which feel worse before bleeding
- *Mercurius* for women aggravated by hot and cold, by sweating, worse at night, and who are awakened by night sweats
- *Phosphorus* for hot flashes from any emotional response
- *Pulsatilla* for the woman who is warm-blooded and aggravated by heat; may sweat more on one side of her body

- *Sepia* for women who tend to be chilly but sweat from hot flashes, worse at night
- *Sanguinaria* for women with hot hands and feet, flushes, and who burn red in their cheeks
- *Sulfur* for the woman who sweats profusely but loves the smell of her own body odor
- *Tuberculinum* for night sweats and flushes with perspiration during the day
- *Valeriana* for flushes accompanied by heat and insomnia

Cooling Herbs

- *Black Cohosh:* 20 drops of tincture three times a day helps to relieve hot flashes, irritability, and some sleep disturbances.
- *Chaste Tree, Vitex:* 10 to 20 drops taken three or four times a day to reduce hot flashes—considered a general nourishing tonic for the menopausal woman
- *Chickweed:* 20 drops two to three times a day to reduce hot flashes in severity and frequency
- *Elder Flower:* 20 drops as often as needed to help with night sweats and hot flashes
- *Nettle Tea:* drink freely to help support adrenals
- *Violet:* drink as a tea throughout your day for heat relief

Other Helpful Suggestions

What to Wear: It is important to feel good about how you present yourself to the world. Maintain a style reflective of your authentic self. Dress in layers of natural fibers. Be prepared to peel off layers and still meet the demands of your workplace or daily activity.

How to Keep Your Bed: Adapt your bed to accommodate night sweats with natural-fiber bedding that breathes with you. Synthetic bedding increases night sweats, as do nylon or polyester nightgowns or pajamas. As you dress in layers, take a similar consideration for your bed. Make up your bedding with layers you can peel off and add on.

Cooling Meditation: Try a cooling meditation to start and end your day. Mentally go there when you feel a hot flash coming on. Slow your breathing to a gentle relaxed pace. Imagine yourself sitting in a cool pool of fresh clear water. Above you a waterfall cascades down, filling the top of your head with its pure refreshing coolness. Let the water flow into the top of your head, through your face, down your throat, through your chest, down your arms, through your torso to your feet. Imagine you're breathing in the scent of spring water. Hear the sound of the water washing over your body. Feel refreshed.

Get Adequate Rest: If your lifestyle allows you to take a nap during the day or to take time out to rest, do so. Set aside fifteen minutes, half an hour, or an hour in the mid- to late afternoon when your energy takes a dive. Pause with a relaxing cup of tea and take a breather.

Exercise, Move Your Body: Find a form of movement that increases your endorphins and feels good. Try swimming if it's an option and you enjoy it; swimming is an excellent exercise that cools as well. Water yoga and yoga are also relaxing. Exercise is a remedy for fatigue and hot flashes. If you feel too tired to exercise, take a walk outdoors and see if your energy level increases, even just a little.

Nurture Stressed Systems: Support your liver and adrenals with nutritionals, herbs, and acupuncture. Work with lowering your response to your stress load, and decrease your stress factors wherever possible. Refer to the stress reduction sections in Chapters 3, 7, and 9.

MY FACE IS FALLING . . . MY BREASTS ARE SAGGING, OH NO!

Beyond vanity, our skin tone, muscle tone, heart and joint integrity, and bone density all rely on hormonal balance. When our body feels intact, functions normally, and feels less fragile, we relax, become less afraid of falling apart, and focus on what stirs our spirit, makes us feel alive.

Shevon's tale of woe, age forty-two

As a professional performer at forty-two, Shevon not only felt plagued by the sudden onslaught of the usual menopausal symptoms of hot flashes, night sweats, and vaginal dryness, but she also complained, "My face is falling." When we first began working together, she had developed irregular cycles and some hair loss. Her gynecologist had given her Premarin and Provera. After one and a half weeks of feeling anxious, fatigued, and losing her memory and her libido, she stopped taking the synthetic HRT.

Compounded phytogenic natural progesterone alone resolved her symptoms for twenty-two months, and then her hormones shifted. Her estrogen levels began to decline. Now, four years later, her formula includes 5 mg of biestrogen, 100 mg of progesterone, and 5 mg of DHEA taken in a capsule twice a day. Applying progesterone cream to the face infuses nourishment directly into the skin desperate for the nutrients normally supplied by our own hormones. Once we lose the ability to produce enough of these precious nutrients, we can begin to shrivel up like prunes. Shevon refused to acquiesce to being a prune-face and allow her career to fade away as well. "Beauty may be only skin deep," she remarked. "But I'm not about to lose my skin—not yet!"

Progesterone, in a 10 percent cream, can be massaged daily into skin areas that show hormonal deprivation—face, breasts, arms. There's no need to use a full dosage as long as you're getting adequate hormonal coverage systemically. Just take a fingerful of cream and apply it to your skin as you would any moisturizer. Although progesterone cream is not specifically an antiwrinkle cream, it does soften and smooth the lines of time.

IS THIS A HEART ATTACK?

Hoshi's story, age thirty-six

My heart started pounding so hard and fast, it took my breath away. My husband loaded me into the car. By the time we arrived at the doctor's office my heart felt more normal. The doctor ran an EKG and some blood tests. Every test he did came back normal. The thought that this could be related to menopause never occurred to any of us. It's happened three times since then. All of a sudden my heart starts racing, pounding really hard, and one time it felt like it was doing flip-flops in my chest. My periods have always been irregular, though now they're lighter. And I have noticed that my mouth seems dry all the time.

Hoshi's progesterone levels measured quite low, as did her DHEA, so she started her hormonal support with 100 mg of progesterone and 5 mg of DHEA along with essential fatty acids. Over the next three months her cycle became more regular and her heart quieted. Hoshi started taking a yoga class and practiced regularly at home. She remained on this formula for eighteen months, after which she began experiencing hot flashes and the return of an occasional flip-flop heart irregularity. Her formula was changed with the addition of 1.25 mg of biestrogen; her progesterone and DHEA remained the same, and she took the Chinese herbal formula Bupleurum D for one month.

Six months later her hot flashes returned, along with sleep disturbances.

> *I awaken with a start, feeling almost a panic. I'm soggy between my breasts and my heart races. I've had to make myself calm down, sit up, take some slow deep breaths until it passes.*

Hoshi needed her estrogens increased, so the new prescription became 3.5 mg of biestrogen, and 100 mg of progesterone with additional progesterone and her calcium supplement at bedtime. Her cycles continued to fade away, now happening at four- or five-month intervals. She continues to get regular exercise, eats well, and remains on this hormonal formula without further incidence of heart palpitations, racing, or flip-flop irregularities.

Heart disease in our Western culture remains a continuing issue for men and women both. In addition to taking a balanced compounded phytogenic hormone formula, Hoshi began to implement healthier lifestyle changes. Unlike synthetic HRT that could increase blood pressure, increase triglycerides, and increase the risk for strokes and heart attacks, compounded phytogenic hormones nourish and help protect the heart.

ADDITIONAL HEART HEALTH SUPPORT

Regular exercise means that you practice some form of movement on a consistently regular basis for a minimum of twenty minutes, four times a week. Increasing the amount of time you exercise either in duration or in the number of days increases benefits.

Quit smoking. If you smoke five or more cigarettes a day, you increase your risk for heart disease. If there is heart disease in your immediate family—parents, siblings, and grandparents—to smoke at all invites the hand of chaos to grip your heart and squeeze. If you have difficulty quitting, switch to a natural, chemical-free cigarette or roll your own and smoke less of the cigarette and less frequently. Even more than the smoke, the unique chemicals and preservatives that each manufacturer of commercial cigarettes infuses into its tobacco can induce cancer, cause addiction, and ensure you will continue to buy a specific brand.

Begin to change your smoking habits. Before you light up, pause and take some slow deep breaths. Do you still need that cigarette, or did the breathing alleviate the urge? Still want the smoke? Take a few puffs, then put the cigarette out. The most damaging part of the cigarette is the part closest to your mouth. If you smoke nonfiltered cigarettes, smoke no more than one-third of it. Set the intention to stop altogether and honor it for your heart, your lungs, your breath, and your loved ones.

Decrease, minimize, or eliminate alcohol intake. An ounce is said to help the heart, more reverses that effect.

Practice compassion and forgiveness. Put away the self-disapproval, criticism, doubt, the nag and all the if-I-had-onlys . . . and practice kindness, compassion, forgiveness, and love with yourself. Pat your heart, alternating hands or with both hands together, and say aloud, "I love my heart." The vibration of patting permeates your chest, carrying the words to the actual organ.

Reduce your stress responses—refer to Chapters 3, 7, and 9 for suggestions.

Eat a low-fat, whole-foods diet—refer to Chapter 5 for suggestions.

Treat hypertension (high blood pressure). This may require medication, but I have seen acupuncture resolve hypertension. Yoga helps lower blood pressure when practiced on a regular basis.

Be orgasmic, not only as a form of release, but for love of self, to nurture, to nourish, to replenish the well of your soul.

Practice heart-opening meditations. Find a meditation during which you can feel the center of your chest expand, relax, and open.

One way to begin is to sit comfortably, close your eyes, and imagine healing rays of light (the color of your choosing or intuition) enter the top of your head, and pour down into your heart chakra in the center of your chest. Let the light settle and pulse with your focused breath. As you inhale, feel the light in your chest draw nourishment from the oxygenated blood circulating through your heart as it pumps. As you exhale, release the toxins from your blood, the negativity, the stress, the tensions, and the responsibilities from your day. Offer gratitude for the opportunity to pause and notice your heart, find peaceful moments and send loving thoughts to your heart and your mind.

Get a massage, once a week, or as often as you can.

Treat yourself to a rose quartz necklace that rests between your breasts over your heart chakra.

Place a drop of *essential rose oil* on the center of your chest and a dot under your nose as an olfactory reminder to focus on your heart in a loving way.

Hug someone with your chest openly expanded, heart to heart, and feel the two hearts beat together. Human contact, touching and being touched, has been scientifically demonstrated as essential for the survival of prematurely born infants. This is true for us all, regardless of whether we are one minute old or one hundred years old.

Hot baths soothe and nurture. Add drops of your favorite scent, light candles, drink something lovely, and return to yourself.

HOMEOPATHIC HEART SUPPORT

- *Cardinorma:* 20 drops three times a day treats cardiac insufficiency, tachycardia, cardiac spasms, circulatory conditions, and increases oxygen utilization.
- *Coro-Calm:* 15–20 drops three times a day of this cardiac sedative will treat tachycardia, disrupted circulatory functions, and pulse abnormalities; it improves oxygenation and calms the nervous response to these conditions.
- *Co-Hypert:* 15–20 drops three times a day to reduce and regulate high blood pressure

OH THEM BONES, THEM BONES

Women are at a four times higher risk than men for the development of osteoporosis, defined by the increased porosity of bones, which causes the bones to degenerate and the bone marrow canals to widen. There are no guarantees that strong healthy bones will not break—that is obvious for anyone who has seen a strong man break his leg. But taking as much action as you can to support optimal bone health may help prevent breakage later in life. As with each system, there is more than one solution to nourish our bones.

Conflicting information suggests that osteoporosis is caused by estrogen and calcium deficiencies. But recent information presented by Drs. John Lee and Jerilyn C. Prior suggests a stronger correlation with progesterone insufficiencies. Women athletes who maintain anovulatory cycles become progesterone deficient yet have sustained normal estrogen levels and have developed osteoporosis. This is directly contrary to the theory of estrogen deficiency. Likewise, women with osteoporosis are not always calcium deficient. Discovering the balance therein and supporting it may help prevent the potential for broken bones. There are many resources and websites that now document these current findings and report effective reversal of osteoporosis with natural progesterone.

Odette's story, age fifty-one

I've been on Premarin and Provera for three years now. My periods stopped seven years ago and my doctor told me to go on HRT to protect my heart and bones. I don't know what good this HRT is doing me—I still get hot flashes, I have mood swings, I'm irritable most of the time, and I have no libido. I want something else.

This was Odette's annual exam and Pap, and I sent her off for a bone densitometry to evaluate the status of her bones, evaluate her risks for osteoporosis, and to see if the synthetic HRT helped her bones. Although there was no known osteoporosis in her family, her mom had breast cancer and heart disease, both of which increased Odette's potential risk while taking synthetic HRT. She immediately stopped taking the HRT and switched to her first compounded phytogenic hormone formula of 2.5 mg of biestrogen with 100 mg of progesterone in an oral capsule, and testosterone cream to assist her libido.

Odette's bone scan showed an alarming decrease in bone mineral density of her lumbar spine and proximal femur, consistent with osteopenia (any decrease in bone mass below the normal), along with in-creased risks of fracture in specific areas. Remember, she had taken Pre-marin and Provera consistently for the previous three years. After reviewing these results, we discussed lifestyle changes and other bone-supportive measures. She agreed to stop smoking, begin a regular exer-cise program that included weight-bearing exercise, work on improving her diet by eating less meat and less dairy, take 1,800 mg of calcium with magnesium and boron, and I increased her biestrogen to 5 mg, with her progesterone remaining at 100 mg. As her diet improved, I lowered her calcium to 1,200 mg.

A bone scan one year later showed improvement in density of every lumbar aspect and some areas of the femoral neck. Odette continues to have some risks for osteoporosis, but less than she did before. She continues to take her compounded hormones, work with the other changes she began, and through her consistent exercise actually is much more athletically inclined than previously. Odette developed a taste for the increased muscle tone and definition that the weight-bearing exercise produced.

> I love it. I feel like a rock. Look at how packed I've become. Being over fifty isn't so bad. Actually, I'm enjoying life more and doing things I never dreamed I would do. I always believed lifting weights was for women who wanted to look like men. But I still feel femi-nine, now I'm a strong feminine, not just in my personality but in my body, too. This is so cool!

Odette will remain mindful of her bones and focus on things that support rather than leach calcium from her bones.

Belinda's experience, age forty-five

> I'm stunned and concerned—to have osteoporosis at my age. I do weight-bearing exercises all the time. I was an athlete most of my life. I don't understand—no one in my family has osteoporosis. And isn't it a disease for old women? My cycles were every twenty-three days until three months ago. I haven't had a period since. I'm hot flashing, the night sweats keep me awake at night, my moods suck, or so my

husband says, and I feel edgy and irritable much of the time. I don't
want to take drugs if I can avoid them.

As Belinda shared her menstrual history, it seemed she often had anovulatory cycles, sustained frequent episodes of PMS, and had most likely
been progesterone deficient for a long time. She started on 5 mg
of biestrogen, 100 mg of progesterone, and 2 mg of testosterone with
100–200 mg of extra progesterone to take at bedtime along with her calcium. Belinda resumed her menses and was happy with how she felt
until seven months later, when her menses started coming closer together, every twenty-one days. She also had a follow-up bone scan,
which showed marked improvement. Because of the increased frequency
of her cycle, I lowered her biestrogen to 3.5 mg, which was fine for the
next eight months.

Belinda started having an occasional night sweat, especially at
the time of her menses, and sleep disturbances, and her libido had declined. Keeping the biestrogen at 3.5 mg, her progesterone at 100 mg,
adding DHEA to her primary systemic cream, and separating the testosterone into a cream for her to apply directly to her clitoral area
made the difference. Over the next year her cycles became light and in-
frequent, until they disappeared and have not returned in the past
twenty-one months. She is now postmenopausal, continues to take her
compounded phytogenic hormones, calcium with extra vitamin D, zinc,
and boron.

WHO IS AT INCREASED RISK FOR OSTEOPOROSIS?

Women who fit into more than two of the following categories are at an
increased risk for osteoporosis.

Alcoholics or those who maintain a consistent alcohol intake
Anorexics/bulimics with sustained periods of no menses
Athletes who skip menses
Birth mothers of more than six children
Coffee drinkers of more than three cups a day
Consistent eaters of processed foods
Diabetics

Drug dependency on: diuretics, anticonvulsants (Dilantin, phenobarbi-
   tal), adrenal corticosteroids, antacids
Drug addicts or abusers of drugs (street drugs or prescriptions)
Fair complexion, light or white skinned
Family history of osteoporosis
Heavy animal protein eaters, daily intake
Hyperthyroid
Inconsistent/negligent with exercise, especially weight bearing
Infertile or have never been pregnant or given birth
Kidney dialysis for disease/failure
Malnourished as children or teenagers or prolonged as an adult
Slender, small frames and bones
Smokers, on a daily basis (not social)
Soda drinkers, daily

ADDITIONAL BONE HEALTH SUPPORT

Try some of these weight-bearing exercises—you may even find you
enjoy them.

Aerobic yoga comes in several forms; find the one that resonates with
   you and your body.
Bicycling out in the fresh air is best, but a stationary bike will do if you
   set the resistance to mimic the open hills.
Bowling, but watch your lower back and dominant arm shoulder—you
   should find some exercise to balance the other side of your body, or
   bowl with both hands down the middle
Climbing stairs counts; at work, take a break and run up and down the
   stairs for fun in the middle of your day.
Dancing, one of my personal favorite forms of movement, definitely counts.
Golfing, if you make sure you walk the course
Hiking, especially the peaks and valleys
Jogging, but nurture your knees
Jumping rope on a forgiving surface to protect your knees
Lovemaking only counts as a weight-bearing exercise if you're acrobatic.
Rowing/paddling a canoe or kayak—the ocean creates more resistance
   than a smooth-water ride, unless you paddle the rapids.
Swimming with fins and webbed gloves

Skiing, especially *cross-country*, and *snowshoeing* give an exceptional workout.

Tai chi looks lightweight, but with focused breath it is powerful, especially when you practice bone breathing.

Tennis; as with any sport that primarily uses your dominant arm, you need to balance your other side.

Trampoline jumping—it can be one of those little ones you stash under your bed or in the corner, or outside with the kids on the one that consumes half your yard

Walking, especially uphill or against resistance; strap on a pair of ankle weights if you don't have any hills.

Weight lifting for both upper and lower body; if you have not done any weight lifting before or for a while, work with a trainer to prevent injury.

DIETARY MEASURES

You should avoid consuming foods that will leach the calcium from your bones. Stay away from:

Caffeine—black tea, coffee, sodas, chocolate
High-protein diets specifically of red meat
Diets high in nonorganic dairy
High intake of acidic foods
Excess sodium (salt) intake

Organic, calcium-rich foods to enjoy include:

Blackstrap molasses
Broccoli
Bok choy
Dark leafy greens
Salmon
Sardines
Seaweeds
Sesame seeds, raw tahini
Soy, tofu
Whey
Yogurt

HOMEOPATHIC REMEDIES

- *BHI Bone* is a combination formula for pain in bones and joints, and it helps increase healing of fractures.
- *Arnica* is the first-line remedy of choice for injuries, including trauma to bones.
- *Asafoetida* helps periosteal and bone pains and inflammation.
- *Aurum* helps with nocturnal bone pain.
- *Eupatorium Perfoliatum* is used when the pain feels like bones are broken or stiff, for excruciating back pain, and to relieve fracture pains.
- *Kali Iodatum* for bones that hurt in the night, sciatica
- *Manganum* for bone pains, especially in the lower extremities and heel, which may cause you to walk awkwardly
- *Picrium Acidum* for back pain, especially spinal, which is worse during mental exertion
- *Syphilinum* for bone pains worse from heat, in skull, arms, and legs, back pain at night

SUPPORTIVE BONE VITAMINS AND MINERALS, NUTRITIONALS

- Boron (3 mg)
- Beta-carotene (10,000–50,000 IU)
- Calcium (800–1,500 mg—too much calcium does not cause kidney stones). Take calcium in chewables, capsules, or liquid for better absorption; hard tablets take longer to break down and dissolve into an absorbable form.
- Vitamin C (1,000–15,000 mg, but not past bowel tolerance)
- Vitamin D (400–800 IU plus 15 minutes or more of sunlight daily)
- EFAs (Essential fatty acids)
- Magnesium (400–700 mg)
- Methylsulfonylmethane, MSM (1 teaspoon a day). Although unproven for osteoporosis prevention or treatment, MSM helps with backaches.
- Phosphorus (800 mg)
- Potassium (2,000–5,000 mg)
- Selenium (15–50 mcg)
- Zinc (10–15 mg)

CHINESE HERBAL FORMULAS

Chase Wind, Penetrate Bone
Essential Yang
Siberian Ginseng

FORGET THEE NOT

Do you find yourself going into another room to retrieve something, but once you get there you haven't a clue what you came to get? Short-term memory loss—you are too young for that one, right? Yet are you writing everything down, carrying a notebook with you wherever you go? One usually does not think of hormones as brain food. But when our hormone levels remain consistently balanced, it seems that we become eloquent once again.

Does estrogen prevent Alzheimer's? Some studies suggest it does. At the time of this writing, no one can say for sure whether it does or not. We do know that natural progesterone plays a significant role in balancing mental and emotional states, and perhaps a greater part in the prevention of mental dysfunction, including Alzheimer's disease. It is also true that when we are in balance—every system, including all our hormones—our brain functions better, becomes more the fine-tuned instrument it is designed to be.

All of the twenty-five emotional and psychological symptoms of perimenopause and menopause (pages 143–145) can play havoc with your mind and state of mental clarity. All of these symptoms can be relieved, including memory loss, by restoring your balance with compounded phytogenic hormones. There comes a point in this process with memory where choice plays a role. Some call it selective memory, which, if done with conscious intent, can be quite manipulative. Beyond that, however, could memory loss be a tool to bring us into the present moment, and make us less focused on events no longer real, the past? To quote the mystic poet Jalal ad-Din ar-Rumi (1207–1273), "Don't grieve what is past. It's over. Never regret what has happened. Let it go. Don't even remember it." As we deepen into growing older, perhaps becoming a little wiser, and with the grace of forgiveness, we can let things go that no longer serve us and choose to focus on our priorities for right now. Our memory can play tricks and alter our perceptions of how we think something may have been. And after we have processed any event, learned what we needed to from an experience, it could be a good thing to let it go and forget it.

BRAIN VITAMINS AND MINERALS

- Vitamin A
- Vitamins B-1, B-6, B-12, B complex
- Vitamin E
- Folic acid
- Niacin
- Pantothenic acid
- Magnesium
- Zinc

OTHER BRAIN SUPPORTS

- *BHI Ginkgo* helps revive weakness and slowness of mental activity and memory loss.
- *Ginseng* improves memory, concentration, mental acuity, and clarity.
- *Sage*—inhaling the fragrance of the essential oil clears your mind.
- *Massaging* your scalp by gently tugging the roots of your hair stimulates the blood supply and circulation to your brain.
- *Meditation* gives your brain a conscious rest and some time off, because even while we sleep, our brain is highly active.
- *Tai chi, yoga, chi gong,* and other such practices clear the mind, enhance mental clarity, and stimulate brain functions.

OTHER NATURAL REMEDIES FOR GENERAL MENOPAUSAL SUPPORT

Currently, there are many products on the market that claim to resolve menopausal symptoms. Some relieve symptoms temporarily but do not effectively address the underlying cause of hormonal deprivation. It is important to nourish yourself in as many ways as possible, but I do see radical sustained relief from the effect of hormonal deficiencies and certain antiaging qualities with consistent usage and adjustments of compounded phytogenic natural hormones. Pure and simple, if you need hormones, *you need hormones.* In each section, you saw alternate natural therapies. They and the following suggestions are meant as an *adjunct* to compounded phytogenic hormone therapy, not as a replacement.

HOMEOPATHIC REMEDIES FOR MULTIPLE MENOPAUSAL SYMPTOMS

For single remedies, refer to the other chapters for details on the actual remedy characteristics. In addition, consider:

- *Ignatia* to help move grief out of your cells, out of the body
- *Lachesis* to assist with hormonal headaches, irritability, jealous rage, and hot flashes
- *Nux Vomica,* known for the irritability factor, helps with night sweats.
- *Pulsatilla* regulates menstrual irregularities, bladder pain and cystitis symptoms, urinary incontinence, and also helps mitigate uterine prolapse.
- *Sanguinaria* helps with headaches and migraines, and facial flushing from hot flashes.

Pekana Homeopathic–Spragyric Medications, a combination formula; dosage: 20 drops three times a day:

- *Klifem* works to regulate menstrual irregularities, to counter the tendency toward obesity in menopause, and helps with hot flashes, night sweats, and breast tenderness.

Heel, Inc., combination formulas; dosage: 10 drops three times a day:

- *BHI Calming* soothes restlessness, irritability, and melancholy, and helps with insomnia.

- *BHI Feminine* for difficult and irregular menses, pelvic pain, vaginal dryness after menses, and hot flashes
- *BHI Liver* helps with liver congestion and related symptoms.
- *Hormeel* helps regulate irregular menstrual cycles, bloating, and nervous irritability.
- *Klimaktheel* helps relieve hot flashes, excessive swelling and edema, headaches, fatigue, and irritability.

HERBAL HELPERS FOR MULTIPLE MENOPAUSAL SYMPTOMS

As previously stated, Chinese herbal formulas are best managed by a skilled practitioner. Here are some formulas by Golden Flower Herbs that have been helpful with more generalized menopausal symptoms.

- *Bupleurum and Tang Kuei* helps with moodiness, irritability, breast distension and tenderness, hot flashes, and regulation of menstrual cycle.
- *Bupleurum plus Dragon Bone and Oyster Shell* can help with hot flashes, insomnia, heart palpitations, restlessness, and urinary symptoms.
- *Cinnamon and Poria* works on blood stagnation in the pelvis, as in uterine fibroids and ovarian cysts, and helps with night sweats.
- *Free and Easy Wanderer* can help regulate irregular cycles, decrease anxiety, restlessness, irritability, and angry outbursts.
- *Heavenly Emperor's Formula* is considered an herbal alternative to tranquilizers and sleeping pills. It assists with forgetfulness and the inability to focus with mental clarity.
- *Rehmannia and Scrophularia* helps with hot flashes, night sweats, and insomnia.
- *Two Immortals* helps with hot flashes, sweating, fatigue, palpitations, and hypertension in menopause.

Note: There are extensive Chinese herbal formulas specific to the variety of symptoms that indicate the need to support your liver.

As the decline of hormones places higher demands on liver function and creates a stress to the liver, women who enter perimenopause with an already stressed liver—from prior disease, excessive use or abuse of drugs and/or alcohol, trauma, or injury—need to support their liver with additional supplements.

There are single herbs believed to alleviate specific menopausal symptoms mentioned throughout. If you find it difficult to drink enough plain water, then find the herbs that nourish you the most and assist with your symptoms, and drink them as teas. Herbal teas count as water. For more extensive herbal information, refer to *New Menopausal Years: The Wise Woman Way,* by Susun S. Weed.

Herbs to Nourish the Liver, the Digestive Tract, and That Help Other Menopausal Disturbances

- *Dandelion:* 10–25 drops before meals relieves digestive distress.
- *Devil's club:* 5–20 drops three times a day evens blood sugar, alleviates constipation, and is beneficial with hot flashes.
- *Fenugreek seeds:* 1 tablespoon per cup of water boiled for ten minutes makes a lovely tea that helps digestion and stabilizes blood sugar.
- *Ginseng:* 5–20 drops three times a day relieves indigestion, reduces fatigue, decreases hot flashes, and can soothe anxiety and depression.
- *Milk thistle:* 175–200 mg one to three times a day nourishes a distressed liver. Some doctors of Oriental medicine say milk thistle is too harsh an herb and prefer combinations of Chinese herbal formulas.

EMOTIONAL SUPPORT

During this transition into the most radical change of your life, connecting with other women who share in the experience helps take the edge off. Knowing you are not alone, especially if you were undergoing a feeling-like-you-are-going-insane phase before you understand that this is caused by menopause, relieves some of the mental and emotional stress factors.

Countless women struggle with the search for adequate support and medical care that is in alignment with their usual nonchemical, organic approach to their health care. Find a physician/practitioner who resonates to your attitudes on health maintenance and who understands compounded phytogenic hormones, or at least holds an open-minded perspective and perhaps is willing to learn. In the Directory (page 281) you will find resources to assist you with referrals to prescribers in your area. When working with your practitioner, it remains important to communicate any hormone-influencing over-the-counter remedy you are taking to better enable accurate assessment of your current hormonal status and to determine the best next step for your optimal support.

RX SUMMARY FOR PERIMENOPAUSE, MENOPAUSE, AND POSTMENOPAUSE

1. Evaluate your hormonal status through either a salivary or twenty-four-hour urine analysis.
2. Chart your cycle, learn your cycle's pattern, and watch the changes. (No need to chart absent cycles if you are already postmenopausal.)
3. Compounded phytogenic hormone therapy, taken twice a day:

   • Progesterone: based on your hormone analysis, or
   • Biestrogen, progesterone, DHEA/testosterone: When formulated for you based on specific deficiencies, symptoms, and analysis to effectively balance your hormones, they will resolve most menopausal symptoms.

   In addition, consider:

For Changes in Cycles
   • Initially try 100 mg of progesterone twice daily for twenty-one days, then off for seven to allow for menses.
   • Progesterone: 100 mg four times a day to stop flooding; dosage can go higher with hemorrhaging under the guidance of your practitioner

For Loss of Libido
   • Testosterone cream: 10 mg per gram, applied to clitoral area twice a day for one month, and as needed afterward

For Insomnia and Sleep Disturbances
   • Progesterone: 100 mg at bedtime

For Loss of Skin Tone

- Progesterone: 10 percent cream applied daily to areas in need

In addition to phytogenic hormone therapy, you may want to consider augmentation with:

4. Balanced nutrition with whole foods; consider dietary suggestions in the sections specific to your symptoms and concerns, plus:

   - Don't eat later than four hours before retiring.
   - Drink plenty of pure water.
   - Limit fluid intake late at night.
   - Limit sweets, especially at night.
   - Avoid caffeine in the evening, or late afternoon.
   - Avoid alcohol if you awaken between two and three A.M.

5. Homeopathic remedies; refer to the area of your concern
6. Herbal helpers; refer to specific sections
7. Balanced multivitamins, minerals, and antioxidants with extra iron, vitamin C, and folic acid in the presence of flooding. Refer to Chapter 4, plus:

   - Calcium (1,200–1,500 mg at bedtime)
   - Magnesium (600–750 mg with calcium)
   - Vitamin B complex (50 mg)
   - Vitamin E (1,200 IU)
   - Iodine (100 mcg)
   - Iron (up to 325 mg three times a day, if anemic)
   - Potassium (up to 6,000 mg)
   - Selenium (15–50 mcg)

8. Rule out thyroid and adrenal dysfunction, treat with glandular support
9. Nutritionals; refer to specific sections
10. Nourish your liver.
11. Move your body; exercise, including your vagina

- Pelvic floor exercises, Kegels
- Sacred spot, also known as G-spot, massage
- Toe-tapping to help open the pelvis

12. Helpful sexual guidebooks include:

    Making Love, by Barry Long

    Healing Love Through the Tao: Cultivating Female Sexual Energy, by
        Mantak and Maneewan Chia

    Taoist Secrets of Love and *The Multi-Orgasmic Man,* both co-
        authored by Mantak Chia (read these with or give them to your
        male partner)

    The Art of Sexual Ecstasy, by Margo Anand

    Sexual Energy and Yoga, by Elizabeth Haich

13. Use natural and nourishing vaginal lubricants.
14. Nourish your creative self and your sensuality.
15. Reduce stress.
16. Support your emotional responses to physical change.
17. Dress comfortably in layers to peel off or add on.
18. Adapt your bedding to your needs.
19. Get adequate rest.
20. Acupuncture
21. Aromatherapy
22. Receive a massage on a regular basis.

PART THREE

TO CUT OR NOT TO CUT, THAT IS THE QUESTION

7

DECREASE YOUR CANCER RISK, INCREASE VITALITY

"Do you know that each woman who is a cancer patient where I work has taken synthetic hormones?" Catrin asked me this question when she came in for her annual exam and Pap smear. The year was 1986 and I had been in private practice, as a women's health care provider, for two and a half years. This question, posed to me by a registered nurse who specialized in oncology, catalyzed my research and my determined quest to discover alternatives for women who need hormonal assistance.

SYNTHETIC HORMONES INCREASE YOUR CANCER RISKS

You might keep in mind that, in the eighties, synthetic hormones were still thought of as a miracle drug. The belief was, and remains so for many practitioners, that if we turn off a woman's own hormonal functioning and dose her with what she needs, she'll be better off. For example, if we prevent ovulation, we prevent ovarian cysts from forming and, indeed, we will prevent cancer. This assumption fails to account for what actually happens on the cellular level when normal hormonal functioning is essentially turned off.

As you may be reading in current literature, there is a significant amount of conflicting information available concerning hormones and cancer. For years it was considered inappropriate, and perhaps even grounds for malpractice, to give a woman synthetic estrogen without progestin if she still had a uterus. Taken without any progestin, known as unopposed estrogen, synthetic estrogen can cause cancer in the endometrium, the lining of the uterus. You may have heard that giving a woman synthetic progestin with her estrogen may increase her risk for breast cancer. What to believe? How does one make discerning choices when the information presented is often conflicting?

The very nature of the interaction between synthetic hormones and the human endocrine system, by shutting down hormonal functioning, increases the risk of cancer, specifically breast, uterine, and possibly ovarian. The human body is not designed to have hormones turned off by chemical or external means. This disrupts the normal physiologic process in any phase of a woman's development throughout her cycles, from the onset of menarche, throughout her childbearing years, independent of pregnancy and childbirth, into the cessation of menses and beyond menopause.

COMPOUNDED PHYTOGENIC HORMONES DECREASE YOUR CANCER RISKS

Compounded phytogenic natural progesterone helps protect our breasts, uterus, and ovaries from developing cancer, particularly if a woman tends to sustain a higher production of estrogen in proportion to her production of progesterone. Rather than suppressing hormone production, we want to augment and support the restoration of balance in the normal ebb and flow of each hormone throughout its cyclic pattern. And once a woman ceases to cycle, supplementing her hormones naturally helps maintain stability and decreases her risk of developing certain cancers.

Years ago I stopped prescribing synthetic hormones for the treatment of any hormonal imbalance. When a woman taking synthetic hormones would come to me for the first time, I would explain why I no longer prescribed her current prescription and clarify her options. In my sense of integrity and conscience, once I discovered compounded phytogenic hormones, I could no longer support the intake of substances that increase a woman's risk of developing some cancers. Most women agree to try these hormones compounded from plant extracts into hormones bioidentical to their own.

As I am a firm believer in choice, I refer those women who choose to continue taking synthetic hormones to practitioners who share their preferences. Make your choices consciously and armed with sufficient information to support your choices. Consider genetic factors that may predispose you to specific increased risks, not out of paranoia but from the perspective of prevention.

For example, if you come from a family of women who have heart disease, you may want to take natural progesterone and estriol to protect your heart rather than synthetic conjugated estrogens and progestin, which can increase your risk for heart disease. If your mother or sister developed breast, ovarian, or uterine cancer, you may want to take compounded phytogenic hormones, primarily progesterone and DHEA, with a conservative approach to estradiol and estriol, to protect your breasts, ovaries, and uterus, as well as taking other supportive, nurturing measures that are life and health enhancing. Although many of these hormonally dependent cancers are considered to be genetically predisposed, I believe we can avert them by maintaining hormonal balance, supporting the immune system, and living in harmony with ourselves, one another, and our ecosystem.

Perhaps the Western way of life is responsible for the rapid rise in cancers, along with the degradation of the environment. Yet every time one person refuses to participate in something that we know potentiates harm, that person effects a positive change, regardless of how small or insignificant it may seem at the time. We always have options, though healthier choices may require you to exert more effort initially as you establish new patterns, habits, and make essential lifestyle changes to enhance your physical integrity, your hormonal balance, your mental and emotional well-being, and your spiritual connection to that which sustains your quintessential self.

SUPPORT YOUR IMMUNE SYSTEM

Feeling healthy and preventing cancer begins with the immune system, our first line of defense on the physical level, and with our mind as we choose how to perceive our sense of self and all aspects of our world. An optimally functioning immune system enables us to eliminate the toxins and abnormal cells that occur throughout a lifetime and can at any time develop into a cancerous and malignant process. Our immune system is designed to eliminate cells that may begin as normal but whose development evolves otherwise. The human body often creates cancer cells on a daily basis, which the well-supported immune function attacks and disposes of without the individual ever knowing a cancerous condition had started.

What supports our immune system to function at its optimum? The maintaining of balance in all aspects of our lives—physically, emotionally, mentally, and spiritually—helps tremendously. Discover what constitutes your own balance right now in your life. Don't compare your current conception of balance to someone else's or even to what may have worked for you a couple of years ago. Most of us change significantly over time and are no longer the same person we were several years ago. When we set an intention and take actions toward satisfying it, we give ourselves the direct message that we value ourselves. I am not suggesting that you set unrealistic goals for yourself. But this is the perfect time to take the opportunity to reevaluate your priorities. Is optimal health one of them?

The fabric of our universe is woven together with the threads of interconnections. So are our physical, emotional, mental, and spiritual bodies. These interconnections work together to create a whole functioning organism. When one of the parts is out of balance, other systems will follow unless balance is restored. Sometimes it takes more than one system to become unbalanced before it gets our attention and we begin to recognize the need for change.

Many women have grown up with the "superwoman complex," thinking they need to handle it all, and often alone. They are often single mothers, or the wives of partners who are rarely home; they manage a job or career, keep the home cozy, raise their children, have a creative focus, volunteer to assist others, go to therapy to work on themselves and become better at all the things they deem to be their job in every area of their lives. Unfortunately, this stresses the immune system, burns out the adrenals, and negates the possibility for others to assist them in this process we call life. We all require good nutrition to fuel the physical body, and nurturing thoughts and sharing love to feed the emotional and spiritual bodies.

If the physical body is in an unhealthy state, it becomes rather difficult to sustain a positive mental attitude. And if the mental or emotional body is sustained at a low or depressed level, the physical body suffers, often through the simple act of neglect. All these interconnections thrive best when balanced.

ELIMINATE TOXINS

Maintaining proper lymph and bowel function is essential in the elimination of toxins, while simultaneously not overloading the body with other toxins. Toxins take many forms in our lives—other than the obvious ones that are added to foods under the guise of additives and preservatives—and they can be cleverly disguised. Relationships in which we stay enmeshed long beyond a healthy duration, praying for changes that never materialize, are emotionally toxic. Falling in love with people's potential rather than seeing who they really are with discernment (not judgment) is also common. When we choose to see what is truth in reality, we can make choices from clarity, not illusion. We want to be well-informed on world events, but the daily television news is often presented from an oppressive, toxic, fear base. Environmental toxins challenge us as well.

Over the next week or so, reflect on the possible toxins that exist in your life. Make an uncensored list of anything that comes to mind that qualifies as a negative factor in your life. It may help to set up categories, such as external sources, environmental sources, work related, relationship related, food sources, emotional sources, mental sources. As you create this list, decide which toxins you can change or eliminate from your life immediately. Next, make a list of everything in your life that nurtures you. And if this list seems rather sparse, add anything you can think of that inspires you.

Can you invite changes into your life that will nourish your body and spirit rather than feed toxicity? If you choose to make these changes, what do you need to do to initiate the process? Take that first step today—for none of us knows what tomorrow may bring.

How we choose to relate to different aspects of our lives remains our choice. Certainly, it appears that many things show up in our reality that we do not consciously choose to invite in. We begin now, in the present moment, and can choose to relate to things from a different point of view. We can choose the path of forgiveness rather than one of holding grudges and anger. Our liver will be pleased. We can choose to see what triggers our negative response as an opportunity to see an aspect of ourselves, delve in deeply, and begin to heal it. Pointing the finger elsewhere to blame others stops, and our mind becomes freer, more compassionate, for everyone, including ourselves. We can choose to accept others for exactly who they present to be at any given moment, trusting that they are doing the best they can, perhaps doing their job well in their eyes, even if we do not like it. When we really see people for who they are and accept them, we no longer hold on to a longing for them to be different, regardless of whether we choose to remain in their lives. Immediately, we sustain more energy within ourselves for whatever is needed, and our emotions cease to do the battle of trying to conjure a methodology to coerce the circumstances into what we think they ought to be, rather than what is.

Often our minds act out with wild thoughts, judgmental and demanding, just like the behavior often demonstrated by a rebellious child. Can we relate to the child who challenges us in countless ways with compassion, with understanding and forgiveness? Can we bring that same understanding to our mind when it tells us negative things? The path of forgiveness, compassion, and understanding begins with oneself. There are many pathways to finding peace inside oneself. Take the time to discover what works for you at this time in your life.

How does all this relate to supporting our immune system? As we eliminate negative stress factors where, how, and when we have the ability, our hearts become lighter, our minds freer. We become more in balance emotionally, mentally, and spiritually. Essentially, we remove many of the obstacles that interfere with our immune system's ability to serve the physical body as it is intended to do. Eliminating toxins, reestablishing an internal harmony that nourishes an inner peace, helps to restore our sense of well-being and energy for the wholeness of life.

REDUCE YOUR RESPONSE TO STRESS

Reducing the stress in life requires, at the very least, that we downgrade our response to it. There always seems to be stress in our lives, much of which feels out of our control. The following list contains simple ways to decrease the effects stress has on you each day.

- Begin this moment anew; don't resurrect anything from the past or project into the future. We begin now, as long as we choose to—herein lies freedom.

- Find gratitude in whatever is happening right now. Many of life's gifts come in rather strange and initially unrecognizable packages.

- Bring your time with yourself and others into balance. Either take at least one hour a day for solitude or, if you spend most of your time alone, make daily time to commune with others.

- Open your day with prayer, meditation, contemplation, and gratitude. Close it this way as well.

- Don't eat in a hurry. If you do not have the time or energy to eat and enjoy your meal right now, have a protein drink and save the savoring for later when you can make the time.

- Cherish your connections with people who love and accept you exactly as you are. Take good care of these precious friendships.

- Avoid repetitive, close, and intimate contact with people who focus on the negative.

- Remove relationships that have a toxic effect on you or any aspect of your life. Hold unconditional love for the person, not for the relationship, their personality, or their pattern of dysfunctional or toxic behavior. Staying in a toxic relationship is like enabling alcoholics, excusing their drinking. You may still love them, but you cannot fix them or realize their potential for them.

- Take slow deep breaths and press the inner pause button whenever you need to take a moment to reevaluate your thoughts, reactions, and feelings.

- Remember, everything takes longer than we think it will; set reasonable schedules. Give yourself an additional half hour for some of the little things, or an extra day when you need it.

- Attempt to create deadlines you can manage without driving yourself and everyone else in your life crazy.

- When you fly to another time zone, set your watch to that time soon after you settle into your seat. Don't think again about the time differential, lost or gained, if you want to alleviate jet lag and decrease stress that is related to time perception.

- Drink lots of pure water, one to two liters a day.

- Rather than trying to become someone or always doing something, just be—be you with you.

- Surround yourself with things you love, things that inspire you, delight your senses, and help you feel content when you are near them, at home or at work.
- Simplify your life wherever, whenever, and however you can.
- Move your body: yoga, tai chi, dance, walk, skip, run, swim, skate, jump up and down, stretch, twist, spin, wiggle, and have some fun with it.
- Laugh as often as you can; call it out of your belly.
- Discover what nurtures your soul and practice it for at least ten minutes a day.
- Spend time in nature, feel the grass with your bare feet, commune with the trees, the rocks, the land, and let them feed you with their grounded strength and their own lines of time.
- Turn the ringer of your telephone off anytime you don't feel like talking, regardless of who may be calling, and especially during meals. Let your voice mail or machine answer for you.
- Treat yourself with kindness, compassion, truth, forgiveness, respect, and love.
- Discover what pleases you and please yourself.
- Make time and space in your day for silence.
- Nourish your creative energy.
- Never let your passion scare you, and if it does, pause to see what really evokes your fear.
- Beauty is internal. The outer echoes the inner. Cultivate your inner beauty and let her shine.
- Goals often mislead and deceive. The unaimed arrow never misses and sometimes finds a much sweeter mark. So stop trying to plan everything. Do things really turn out the way you think they will?
- All problems are simply challenges awaiting a new point of view.
- Question yourself honestly when you find yourself thinking or saying "But it's always/forever/never/probably/totally/definitely/absolutely . . ." Is it true that *it* is *always* or *never*? These words usually reinforce a negative mind-set. Try dropping the definitive adverbs and adjectives. Consider replacement words if you need a descriptive—"it seems, it appears, possibly . . ."
- Stop worrying. Worrying is praying for what you do not want. No worries.

- Don't take *it* personally. If *it* truly feels personal, look to see what is being mirrored for you and explore inside yourself—is *it* accurate?
- Draw the line of boundaries with discernment and choice, not judgmental behavior.
- It is okay to say no, and you do not need to wait for the diagnosis of cancer to begin to say no and not feel guilty.
- Choose the words you speak to be the closest to the truth as you know it to be in your heart, in that moment.
- Share love every day, even if it's in your thoughts and you send love telepathically. Look into someone's eyes, feel your connections, and tell them you love them without expecting anything in return.
- Forgive someone right now. Accept whatever he or she did even though you did not like it or agree with it.
- Expectations breed discontent. Give up your expectations and embrace the moment, the mystery.
- Look for beauty in anything.
- Offer only that which you are really able to fulfill. Empty promises carry a heavy burden. Better not to offer, and if it works out, do it because you truly want to and can.
- Keep something juicy, inspiring, or interesting to read with you at all times.
- Take one day a week for you, for your regeneration cycle.
- Discover yourself, the person you are, undefined by what you do for a living or the expectations of others, real or imaginary. "To thine own self be true" only happens when you inquire into just who you really are and live to your fullest.
- Remember, you are not your job, or your home, or your car, or your children, husband, lover, friends, or the lack of any of these.
- Listen to your inner guidance and follow through with actions based on what she tells you. When we do not listen to our inner voice, we hurt ourselves.
- Do not deny or suppress your shadow side; take a mental health day off to sit with her. Hear her story and give her a healthy form of expression. Delving into and dancing with your shadow is self-revealing; it shows you sources of anger, defeat, sorrow, joy, and inspiration, and enables you to access self-forgiveness. Either this, or she may act out when you least expect it. And it may not be pretty.

- It is whatever we tell ourselves it is. When our minds say "It is bad, it is hard, I'm really stressed out," our energy follows our thoughts and we begin to feel bad, tired, or really stressed out. Another way to relate to any scenario is, perhaps: *It just is . . .*

- Slow *it* down. Let *it* go. Be fully present with what *is* and recognize the sacred—for you, in you. Time ceases to exist when we totally immerse ourselves in something. And the cessation of the demands we define in time . . . that is something truly sacred.

- There is no time but now. If *it* is important to you, then do *it* now, say *it* now, or be *it* now. We know not what the morrow may bring.

- Stop trying to satisfy the needs of all whose lives you touch. Allow them to share their gifts with you as well.

IMMUNE-SUPPORTING NUTRITIONALS

In considering the following practical immune-support suggestions, it helps to know what specific modalities work best for you. Think of the times you have taken a nutritional supplement, herb, or remedy. Did you notice any improvement or resolution of a particular issue when you took, for example, an herbal remedy, but you did not feel any different when you took vitamins? Or do you respond rapidly to homeopathy and less so with herbals? The quality of the product influences the experience of effectiveness as well. How quickly do you feel a positive response? Or are you someone who has never tried anything other than commercial products found in a regular pharmacy? I am sharing with you specific modalities that, in my experience as a practitioner, have been significantly successful.

As you read these alternative options, trust your inner guidance, your intuition. If something sounds right to you or you get a clear yes, try it for four to six weeks and observe the effects. When we are addressing more long-term issues and conditions, the response time tends to seem slower than in acute conditions, and a four- to six-week period before noticing change is common. You may find it useful to keep a journal or log of your experience to assist your self-evaluation process. If you do not know the best approach for yourself, it may be a process of elimination. And if you do not experience any change within that time frame, that specific remedy or manufacturer may not be the right one for you.

Homeopathy

Homeopathic approaches to reestablish homeostasis in immune function are often addressed as a constitutional remedy specific to the individual being. Unless you know your constitutional remedy, work with a homeopath with whom you can easily connect and establish an authentic rapport. An effective constitutional workup necessitates you to be honest about who you are, sharing personal and intimate details of how you live your life. The initial interview usually takes a couple of hours.

Enzyme Process formulates combinations that include different homeopathic remedies with glandulars and specific vitamins. Their *Blood Liquezyme* provides nutrients essential for the repair of blood cells. Cleansing the blood of toxins remains one of the first-line defenses of our immune function, along with supporting the lymphatics for adequate drainage of those toxins. Both *Blood* and *Lymph Liquezyme* can be taken as one teaspoon three times a day held under the tongue for a moment before swallowing. For more information on Enzyme Process, go to *www.enzymeprocess.com*.

Colloidal Silver

In the presence of infections and inflammations, colloidal silver helps to further support immune function by acting as a secondary immune system. Take one teaspoon, an average dosage of colloidal silver equaling ten parts per million, three times a day for seven to ten days to boost your immune system and treat the infection. Unlike with antibiotics, if your symptoms resolve within a few days you can discontinue taking colloidal silver. If at any time you feel as if you are coming down with a bug or threat to your immune system, you can initiate the above dosage. If your immune system has been overstressed or compromised for an extended time, after treating the acute problem, take one teaspoon of colloidal silver daily for three to six months.

Over the nine years since it became available in 1993, I have worked with many kinds of colloidal silver. *Silverloid,* by Longevity Formulas, consistently yields the most significant results, in my experience. Colloidal silver has proven itself effective as an antibacterial, antifungal, and antiviral solution. For more information, go to *www.longevity formulas.com/immunity.html#Anchor Antisep 28250.*

Nutritional Supplements

Intended as a nutritional support for immune enhancement, *Beta 1, 3 D Glucan* is a cell wall component of yeast effective in augmenting cellular growth and activity. These vegetable-based capsules are taken on an empty stomach, three times a day. Professional Complementary Health Formulas can be located at *www.professionalformulas.com.*

Also helpful, the *noni plant,* used for generations by South Pacific islanders, enhances immunity by repairing damaged cells on a molecular level. Research on noni and its phytochemicals continues as it has demonstrated anticancer qualities by increasing the effectiveness of white blood cell activity. It can be taken in its liquid juice form or in capsules. Dosages vary depending on the condition. As a general immune support, take one dose a day. A Hawaiian, certified organic source is best.

Olive Leaf Extract: Olive leaf extract has been found to enhance immunity and to act as a natural antiviral approach to many immune-compromising conditions. Recently, many people have successfully used it to treat herpes simplex virus (HSV). The dosage for olive leaf is 500–1,000 mg every six hours, and it is most effective when initiated at the first signs of an infection. For more information go to *www.olive leafextract.com.*

Olivirex, produced by Bio-Botanical Research, Inc., is a combination of olive leaf extract with goldenseal, garlic, St. John's wort, uva ursi, milk thistle, cordyceps, noni, ginseng, white willow, dandelion, and bladder wrack. Taking one or two capsules three times a day helps inhibit the growth of bacteria, fungi, and parasites while promoting the removal of these pathogens and their waste by-products. For more information, go to *www.biobotanicalresearch.com.* It can also be ordered along with your compounded hormone prescription through Women's International Pharmacy.

Ume Concentrate/Plum Extract, a concentrate extracted from the Japanese umeboshi plum, enhances our ability to increase the absorption of other nutrients we take in. Ume adjusts the pH balance by decreasing acidity and increasing alkalinity. Take a pea-size amount of the concentrate dissolved in one-quarter cup of warm water and drink it fifteen minutes before meals. For more information go to *www.eden foods.com/.*

Rain-Forest Herbals: There are now many herbals grown in virgin soil in the rain forests, which are considered to contain the planet's highest concentration of life energy. Consider herbal support from the highest-quality botanicals harvested using methods that are respectful of the local environment, ecology, and inhabitants. One such company is Amazon Herb Co., *www.rainforestbio.com/amazonherb/*. They have several formulas that work with enhancing immune function. *Arcozon* strengthens your body's defenses, *Environzon* purifies the body, and *Una de gato* supports immune functions. The average dosage is one dropperful of a tincture three times a day. This dosage can be doubled when assisting acute problems.

Chinese Herbs: Chinese herbals are most effective when prescribed by an acupuncturist/herbalist who understands your constitution and the nature of the herbs. These herbs are formulated to build or replenish chi or qi, and to nourish and tonify the blood and specific organs that are weak or deficient. Because many formulas are specific to conditions and contraindicated to certain symptoms, I encourage you to consult a qualified practitioner. A good resource is Golden Flower Chinese Herbs, found at *www.gfherbs.com/*.

Here are a few formulas to consider:

- *Astragalus and Ligustrum Formula* to support normal qi
- *Ginseng Nourishing Formula* for qi and blood deficiency, recovery from a long illness
- *Intestinal Fungus Formula* for intestinal heat toxins and dampness, as well as candidiasis
- *Jade Screen and Xanthium Formula* for allergies and to tonify
- *Minor Bupleurum Formula* to support normal qi
- *Siberian Ginseng* for stress, kidney and liver deficiency, dampness, and stagnation

Vitamins: In addition to finding the brand of vitamin and mineral supplements you can absorb and utilize well, extra B vitamins, antioxidants, and higher dosages of vitamin C remain important to augment and optimize your immune functioning. Whenever you need to actively fight off an invading pathogen, increasing vitamin C intake *up to bowel tolerance* expedites the process. The term *up to bowel tolerance* means increasing the dosage of vitamin C in increments of 500–1,000 mg at a time until diarrhea has been induced. Then decrease the dosage to the next dosage below the amount that caused the diarrhea. If you are highly sensitive, increase your dosage by 500 mg per dose. It is safe to start with 1,000 mg taken orally three or four times a day, increasing to bowel tolerance, which for some people can be at least 10,000 mg a day. We tolerate much higher dosages of intravenous vitamin C than we can take in orally. Please refer to the section on vitamins and minerals for PMS for more details on the specific vitamins.

8

BREAST LUMPS

BREAST TOUR

Women's breasts are composed of lobes of glandular tissue, fifteen to twenty primary sections in each breast, separated from one another by many smaller lobules at the end of which are clusters of tiny bulbs. Milk production occurs in these bulbs. And all of these components link through ducts—the thin tubes leading to the nipple. The areola is the darker skin encircling the nipple. Fat cells fill most of the space between the lobules and ducts, which is why our breasts grow larger when we gain weight. A general sense of breast lumpiness is common for most women and does *not* suggest disease.

HORMONES' INTERRELATIONSHIP WITH BREASTS

As is evident in any woman who has been pregnant, breasts undergo dramatic transformations with the elevation and shifting of hormones. Our ever-changing hormones interact with our breasts cyclically as well. A woman may experience swelling, enlargement, and a lumpy condition, as well as pain and tenderness, each month between ovulation and the onset of bleeding. Once she begins to bleed, her breasts return to normal. These fluctuations are a result of changing levels of progesterone and reflect the need to readjust levels of progesterone to reestablish a balanced ratio to estrogens.

BENIGN BREAST CONDITIONS

Throughout a woman's life, breasts endure many changes. If you ever become pregnant, regardless of whether you carry to term, you will notice significant variations in the size and the texture of your breasts. In fact, every woman of childbearing age, the time in our lives when our breasts are the most glandular and hormonally reactive, is likely to develop noncancerous breast conditions. These benign, noncancerous conditions do not evolve into a malignant process and do not increase the risk of developing cancer at a future date, but they do manifest as generalized breast changes, infections or inflammations, nipple discharge, or a distinct and usually solitary lump. Eighty percent of all breast conditions actually biopsied prove to be benign, and many more breasts never see the tip of a needle or surgical blade because the condition disappears before the woman sees a surgeon.

Benign breast conditions, as well as certain breast cancers, correlate with an imbalance in the ratio of estrogens to progesterone on the physical level. And from a holistic perspective, I have seen a consistent pattern of imbalance in the woman who has an amazing ability to take care of everyone else, to nurture the many people in her life, but lacks practice in the art of receiving. She is adept at breast-feeding the world but either has little experience in accepting nurturance from others or seems to be unable to allow them to give of themselves to her.

This kind of imbalance resides in the old assumption that our world lacks enough to nurture and sustain each of us. *"I have enough energy and love to take care of others, but by the time I get around to myself, I am just too tired."* Does any of this ring even a little bit true for you? You now have an opportunity to reassess your life, permit yourself to become aware of other choices, and to create new options for how you want to live your life.

FIBROCYSTIC BREASTS

In fibrocystic breasts, breast tissue feels ropelike and has a stringy texture. Most often, this congested breast tissue is more pronounced in the upper outer quadrant of both breasts, though it can be found behind the nipple areas as well. While this is referred to as fibrocystic breast disease, the use of the term *disease* implies pathology, involving a progression of changes in structure and function. Fibrocystic breasts, however, do *not* advance into a disease process, though due to the denseness of the tissue, it is possible for a mass to hide behind the fibrocystic tissue. The fibrocystic condition can be quite uncomfortable for many women, while others may not even notice it.

Caffeine usage, ingesting exogenous estrogens from the meat of hormone-injected animals, and a low progesterone level have all been linked to causing fibrocystic breasts. Eliminating caffeine, particularly coffee, and commercial meats and dairy, and adding a natural progesterone supplement usually resolves the condition within one to three cycles.

Homeopathic Remedies
- *Calcarea Carbonica*
- *Carbo Animalis*
- *Carcinosin*
- *Conium*
- *Phosphorus*
- *Phytolacca*
- *Silica*

Brittney's experience, age thirty-two

> Both of my breasts feel hard as rocks to the touch a week or so before my period starts. They get so tender that I cannot tolerate to be touched by my partner.

Brittney shared this at her annual exam not realizing that she could have addressed her pain sooner. She thought she simply had to endure this uncomfortable condition every month and was surprised to learn she could treat it naturally. At thirty-two years old, Brittney was a single mother of one child, had been divorced, and survived two other challenging relationships. She worked in a high-stress profession and found little time alone, for herself, except in sleep. During her visit she confessed:

> I don't want to mother my lover, too. One child is enough. Because he works hard all day, making responsible decisions, he wants me to

make all the decisions about what to eat for dinner, what to do in the evenings we spend together, where to go on holiday, about anything concerning the two of us together. But I am required to make intense decisions all day long as well. It seems like the men I attract into my life just want me to take care of them. And I must admit, I probably do too good a job of it. No wonder I resent him sucking on my breasts when we make love. Maybe I don't deserve a man who can take care of himself, let alone take care of me.

Brittney reached the realization, through flowing tears, that she needed to make some changes in her relationship as well as treat her fibrocystic breast condition. After two months of a 10 percent progesterone cream twice a day from midcycle to her menses, cutting out coffee, and taking homeopathic Silica 200C four times a day the week before her period, her breast tenderness and the fibrous, rocklike consistency of her breast tissue vanished.

CYSTS

Common among women in their early thirties through their fifties are fluid-filled sacs, cysts, that occur in the breast singularly or in multiples. Cysts range in size from too tiny to detect on exam to the size of a walnut. Affected by our cycles, cysts may enlarge, becoming quite tender or painful, just before menses. Not all cysts require a fine-needle aspiration. Many can be treated with a combination of warm ginger compresses and natural progesterone therapy.

Becca's experience, age twenty-four

There's a lump in my right breast. I noticed it before my period and I thought it might just go away. It got bigger and more painful the closer I came to my period and then after I started bleeding, it seemed to get a little smaller. But it did not go away. I'm a little scared. Is it cancer? No one in my family has had breast cancer. How can one day my breast be normal and the next day there's a lump?

Becca trembled as she spoke to me. We talked briefly about what she experienced during her cycle and the unlikelihood for cancer to spontaneously become smaller simply because her menses had started. Upon exam, an encapsulated cyst, round with smooth borders and a fluidy feeling, about the size of a grape, was found fairly close to the surface of her breast. Becca decided she wanted to try a noninvasive approach first, and if it did not cure it, she would then have it aspirated with a needle.

For one week, Becca applied warm ginger compresses to the cyst twice a day. Reluctantly, she gave up coffee, but only completely for that one week. After she was convinced the cyst was almost gone, she allowed herself a cup of coffee each morning, but switched to using organic beans and organic milk. She also took 100 mg of progesterone twice a day, in sublingual drops, from midcycle until the onset of her menses. Each day she massaged a couple of the drops onto the cyst. When Becca's next cycle began, she called to tell me that the cyst had completely vanished and she was having the best cycle she could remember—no PMS, no cramps, and her bleeding seemed less heavy.

FIBROADENOMAS

Brighid's experience, age twenty-six

> I awoke to find a firm, round lump in my right breast. My heart started racing as I went to a mirror to get a good look at it. It was not there when I went to bed the night before. How could a lump that I can see and feel erupt overnight? It was about an inch in diameter and clearly poking out. I went to work as usual in the OR—I'm a scrub nurse—and on a break I showed it to one of the docs I work with, who scheduled me for surgery the following week.

Upon further probing, Brighid, who at twenty-six preferred to keep her breast unscarred, wanted to explore an option other than surgery. As a nurse, she recognized that a freely mobile lump with clearly defined, smooth round borders was not likely to be cancer. The painless, rubbery lump in her breast was a fibroadenoma, a solid, round, benign tumor consisting of structural and glandular tissue. Fibroadenomas, usually found by the woman herself, are the most common type of breast lump, especially in women in their late teens into their mid-twenties. If a fibroadenoma develops during pregnancy and/or nursing, it will likely enlarge.

Brighid canceled the surgery because, after taking 200 mg of progesterone and applying a warm ginger compress for seven days, the fibroadenoma disappeared. (It is also possible for a fibroadenoma to disappear spontaneously.) She discontinued the progesterone after two months without further incidence of the fibroadenoma returning and no longer needed progesterone therapy until ten years later, when her cycles became irregular while she was going through a stressful time.

NIPPLE DISCHARGE

Any woman can experience discharge from her nipples, and this does not necessarily indicate the presence of disease. Often the liquid contained in nipple discharge is composed of fat cells. A milky-appearing secretion, which tends to be more opaque in consistency, can have many causes, such as a thyroid malfunction or a side effect from medications. Nipple discharge can also be a side effect of taking birth control pills, sedatives, or tranquilizers. As our breasts are glandular, it is not unusual for a woman to have secretions from the breast. And if a disease causes a discharge from your nipple, it is more likely to be *noncancerous*, or benign.

A woman who stopped nursing her baby ten years ago can extract a milky-looking discharge if she squeezes her nipples with enough oomph. Not all nipple discharge is galactorrhea, the continuation of lactation after nursing has been discontinued. Galactorrhea can be treated homeopathically, herbally with sage tea, and/or with natural progesterone.

Homeopathic Remedies
• *Calcarea Carbonica*
• *Pulsatilla*

In the presence of a cyst, the color of the fluid can even appear black-looking, though more transparent than when it's milky. During a breast infection or inflammation, the fluid may have a greenish tinge, or actually resemble pus. The fluid can be expressed onto a slide and viewed under a microscope to identify its cellular nature. Certainly, anytime there's discharge, it's wise to check it out, particularly if blood is easily expressed with little applied pressure. It's easy to see how a little blood vessel might break and leak a trace of blood into the discharge if a nipple is squeezed hard enough, which happens when a woman who experiences nipple discharge works really hard to express the secretions. It should not be necessary to work at it to determine if there's a discharge, and the action can create localized trauma. The discharge is either present, and easily expressed with little or no effort, or it is not.

MASTITIS

This breast inflammation, most commonly experienced in lactating women, can occur at any age. Usually bacteria enter the breast through a portal in the nipple, either through a crack or abrasion, and induce infection beginning in a lobule.

Postpartum mastitis, caused by a blocked milk duct where the milk collects and pools, produces marked inflammation and occurs after giving birth. If discovered early, when the breast first becomes noticeably warm or hot to the touch, tender or actually painful, and lumpy, warm ginger compresses and homeopathic remedies can negate the need for antibiotics and resolve this very distressing condition quickly.

The new mother is encouraged to continue nursing her babe to help prevent the inflammation from worsening and turning into an abscess. Once advanced to a more progressed stage, apparent by the exquisite pain—pain too acute to nurse the baby from that side—antibiotics are indicated. The duration of infection will be shorter by taking the correct homeopathic remedy and using the ginger compresses, even if antibiotics become necessary. Many new mothers become progesterone deficient after giving birth and need supplemental support to prevent numerous other postpartum conditions.

Natural progesterone does not cure mastitis once it develops. However, it does help prevent mastitis from arising. Mastitis in a nonlactating woman, which is not particularly common, is treated the same as postpartum mastitis with the exception of the breast-feeding. Typically, mastitis develops in one breast, not both.

The earliest sign of any mastitis is marked by a triangular flush on the skin and an elevation of body temperature, eventually giving rise to a high fever and a rapid pulse rate.

- *Cystic mastitis* feels knobby or nodular, due to the formation of multiple cysts.
- *Interstitial mastitis* is an inflammation of the connective tissue.

- *Parenchymatous mastitis* is the inflammation of the breast's secreting tissue.
- *Puerperal mastitis* occurs toward the end of lactation, usually as the baby nurses less, accompanied by painful engorgement of milk and the formation of pus that can develop into an abscess.
- *Stagnation mastitis* is marked by painful distension, a caked breast, and occurs early in lactation.

For additional remedy details, see the homeopathic section in Nonsurgical Treatment for Benign Breast Conditions (page 233).

Homeopathic Remedies
- *Belladonna* for right-sided breast infections, when there is great tenderness, heat, and inflammation
- *Bryonia*
- *Hepar Sulphur*
- *Phellandrium*
- *Phytolacca*
- *Pulsatilla*

BREAST ABSCESS

An abscess found in any part of the body, defined by the formation of a localized collection of pus, and particularly when in the breast, is very painful with acute inflammation. Traditionally, this has been treated by surgically removing the abscess or draining the pus through a needle or surgical incision. Hepar Sulphur is an excellent remedy for a breast abscess, as is Phytolacca. I have seen breast abscesses cured without surgical intervention through the aggressive combination of warm ginger compresses, homeopathy, colloidal silver, and other immune-system boosters.

Homeopathic Remedies
- *Carbo Animalis*
- *Hepar Sulphur*
- *Phytolacca*
- *Silica*

MAMMARY DUCT ECTASIA

As a woman's hormones shift out of balance with the approach of the menopausal process, the ducts beneath the nipple may become inflamed and sometimes clogged. Painful mammary duct ectasia produces a thick, sticky, grayish to green nipple discharge. Treatment with warm ginger compresses, hormone and immune support, and sometimes homeo-pathic augmentation, initiated as soon as the condition is discovered, avoids the need for antibiotics or the surgical removal of the duct.

Brenda's story, age forty-six

> My period began two days ago, and with it my right breast suddenly became swollen, the skin looks quite red, and it really hurts. Actu-ally, my other breast is a bit tender as well. I could not sleep much last night because of the pain, and I guess I worried all night.

At forty-six, Brenda was in the early stages of perimenopause when she developed mammary duct ectasia. This condition disappeared com-pletely within six days of beginning treatment using warm ginger com-presses twice a day for twenty minutes, boosting her immune function with 2,000 mg of vitamin C three times a day, taking other antioxidants, and making a hormonal adjustment to include a low dose of 1 mg of biestrogen, 100 mg of progesterone, and 5 mg of DHEA taken twice a day. She did not need surgical intervention or antibiotics.

FAT NECROSIS

Typically, fat necrosis—a painless, round, firm lump—develops in women exhibiting obesity who also have very large breasts. Damaged and disintegrating fatty tissue forms these lumps, sometimes as a reac-tion to a bruise or bump to her breast. The incident of trauma may have been so insignificant that the woman does not remember bumping or bruising herself. The skin surrounding the lump can look discolored or reddened. Surgical removal is recommended because fat necrosis resem-bles and can be mistaken for breast cancer.

While awaiting removal of the lump, it is reasonable and safe to try the suggested treatments of compounded phytogenic natural progesterone, ginger compresses, immune support, self-nurturance, and homeopathic remedies. If the lump begins to reduce in size, you may want to continue the treatment for up to one month. If no size reduction is apparent, removal can provide diagnostic clarity and peace of mind.

SCLEROSING ADENOSIS

Breast pain caused by an excessive growth of the tissues in the breast's lobules, called sclerosing adenosis, can also produce lumps, and they may show up on mammography as calcifications, small calcium deposits in the breast tissue. Because this condition is difficult to distinguish from breast cancer, taking a biopsy clarifies the diagnosis. However, each of the nonsurgical treatment suggestions found at the end of the chapter may help diminish the lumps and assist your body in breaking down the calcifications and excreting them as toxins.

INTRADUCTAL PAPILLOMAS

A small wartlike growth that projects into the breast duct near the nipple, an intraductal papilloma produces one of the most common sources of a bloody or sticky nipple discharge. This benign breast condition, when it presents with an isolated papilloma, affects women as they evolve closer to menopause.

The sensitive papilloma bleeds easily when the nipple area becomes bruised or is slightly jolted. Younger women who develop this condition are more likely to have more than one papilloma and to have them in both breasts. They may find the lump in the nipple area, which then reveals nipple discharge. In the presence of lumps, the recommendation is to remove the papilloma. While awaiting a date with the surgeon, it is safe to consider and use nonsurgical treatments—warm ginger compresses, immune support, and hormonal balance with emphasis on phytogenic progesterone. If the papilloma disappears with this noninvasive approach, there is nothing to surgically remove nor is there a need to prove that the papilloma is benign. Refer to the nonsurgical treatments at the end of the chapter.

DO BENIGN BREAST CONDITIONS BECOME BREAST CANCER?

The answer is *no*.

Most benign breast changes and conditions do *not* increase a woman's risk for developing breast cancer. Studies suggest that hyperplasia, an excessive growth of cells, found in conditions such as intraductal papilloma and sclerosing adenosis, may *slightly* increase the risk of developing breast cancer. In the presence of atypical (abnormal) cells and hyperplasia, there is a moderate increase of breast cancer risk.

Remember, 80 percent of the breast conditions that are actually sampled through a biopsy are benign and not cancer. And not every lump remains present long enough to require a biopsy. It is a rare event for breast cancer to spontaneously disappear. If you have a lump in your breast, evaluate it with someone who has skilled hands you trust, and whose opinion you respect. If your lump goes away, with or without the following treatment, it is highly unlikely that it could be malignant.

NONSURGICAL TREATMENTS FOR BENIGN BREAST CONDITIONS

NATURAL PROGESTERONE THERAPY

Although many surgeons believe it is wise to remove a fibroadenoma, cyst, abscess, intraductal papilloma, sclerosing adenosis, or mammary duct ectasia to prove it benign or simply to get it out, many of these benign breast conditions do resolve with nonsurgical treatments. The compounded phytogenic natural progesterone, taken at a dose of 100 mg twice a day, stabilizes your hormonal balance of progesterone to estrogen. Sublingual or transdermal absorption is quickly effective for most women. A 10 percent progesterone cream applied every twelve hours, some of which should be gently massaged directly on the affected area with the remaining dosage applied to rotated locations, for twenty-one days of your cycle also helps.

If you do not have regular cycles, try using it for three weeks, then not using it for one week. The progesterone cream or progesterone dissolved in a vegetable oil will be absorbed into the localized affected area and help to balance the glandular aspect in your breast. If you choose to evaluate your hormone levels before initiating any treatment, adjust your dosage accordingly.

HOMEOPATHY FOR BREAST CONDITIONS

A note on the dosage of homeopathic remedies: Unlike allopathic drugs, the remedy can be discontinued with resolution of symptoms rather than when you have "completed the course." The average dosage includes taking a 30C or 200C potency two to four times a day, or a 1M potency every twelve hours for three dosages. Some homeopaths will dose the person once a week. You may want to consult with your homeopath to assess the correct remedy, potency, and dosage for your condition.

- *Belladonna* is for the woman who experiences a sudden onset of mastitis, often accompanied by high fever and deep redness to the affected area. Her breast is hot to the touch—almost the feeling of being scalded—and marked with much inflammation. There is significant tenderness with an intense throbbing or pulsing sensation.
- *Bryonia* is appropriate for a woman who is quite irritable when she develops mastitis: The fever comes on slowly, her condition worsens over several days, her breast becomes hard and hot, and the inflammation occurs more often in the right breast.
- *Calcarea Carbonica* is for breasts that swell and sometimes feel hot. If a woman's milk supply was abundant while nursing, may at times have been disagreeable to her baby, and continues to be excessive after weaning, galactorrhea may be present.
- *Carbo Animalis* is used for fibrocystic breasts, breast abscesses, and breast tumors or breast cysts that tend to emerge on her left side.
- *Carcinosin* is useful in the presence of painful, swollen premenstrual breasts, and it helps fibrocystic breasts.
- *Conium,* one of the main remedies to help resist malignant and premalignant conditions, has been used to help treat breast cancer, often with axillary lymph node involvement, and to treat cyclic cystic breast conditions.
- *Lac Caninum* is appropriate for the woman who, before her menses, is likely to develop painful, swollen breasts that worsen if she is bumped or jolted.
- *Hepar Sulphur* is for the woman extremely sensitive to pain, especially

as the pain increases her sense of vulnerability, as she develops mastitis and/or a breast abscess.

- *Phellandrium* is mainly used in the treatment of mastitis. There can be significant pain in her right breast with a stitching pain extending to her back. The woman may experience painful nipples during nursing.
- *Phosphorus* is a good remedy for fibrocystic breasts.
- *Phytolacca* is a glandular-focused remedy that assists with fibrocystic breasts, characterized by painful breasts before and during menses, and painful benign breast lumps. It has also been known to palliate breast cancer, though not cure the disease itself. Infections occur in the left breast with intense pain from nursing that radiates throughout the entire body.
- *Pulsatilla* treats galactorrhea, mastitis, and fibrocystic breasts.
- *Silica* is recommended for the nursing mother who develops mastitis. She can have a tendency toward fibrocystic breasts. Silica also treats breast abscesses and nodules.

COMPRESSES AND POULTICES

Ginger Compress

A hot compress—but not so hot that it burns your skin—made from strong fresh gingerroot tea will not only feel soothing but also help your body begin to break down the cellular components of the condition and assist the body in eliminating the toxins. Take a 2-inch or so piece of fresh gingerroot and either slice it thinly or grate it with a ginger grater. Keeping the lid on tightly, steep this in one pint of boiled water and allow it to cool to the warmest temperature comfortable to your touch. Now find a cozy, relaxing place to lie down for twenty minutes undisturbed. Take the pot of ginger tea, lid secured to keep it hot, and place it within easy reach.

There are various ways to create the compress. One is to simply place a clean cloth into the tea, squeeze out the excess liquid, and fold it to the right size to completely cover your breast condition. You can place a hot-water bottle on top to help maintain the temperature. Or have a second cloth waiting in the tea and replace the first when it cools down.

Lie down in a comfortable position on your back with pillows propped around you. Your pot of tea sits on the table or stool next to you; all you need to do is move your arm or hand to reach it. Perhaps you have your favorite music on, or maybe you are enveloping yourself in silence. Breathe in the scent of ginger. Where does your mind travel? Do you imagine the tropical jungles where the ginger grows wild? Do fearful thoughts about your body arise? Does your mind wander to the myriad of undone chores you put aside for this brief respite? Inhale the scent of ginger. Take a sip of this hot nectar. Taste it. Let the droplets saturate your tongue before you swallow.

Allow your mind to focus on your breast. Can you feel it from the inside, while you change to a warmer compress? Go inside with your mind's inner vision, your inner knowing, and connect with your breast. Does any particular image arise? Ask this inner knowing, the wisdom of your true self that trusts the course of your existence, if there is anything your breast wishes to communicate to you. Breathe in the scent of the ginger and feel your body relax. As you let go of the day, feel yourself present with you alone and nothing else. If worries arise, be aware of your inner response. Do you go into fear? Can you question the inner wanderings of your mind and investigate what is really true? Do you assume that something bad may be happening? If so, check it out. Make sure you have a clear understanding of your diagnosis, that you have been evaluated by someone whose skills you trust. Or get a second opinion.

Let any form of connection and communication reveal itself. Try not to control it or even grasp a meaning just yet. Just breathe into your breast. Send loving energy into your entire chest area and feel your heart expand. The warm ginger compress rests on the affected area of your breast below the palm of your hand. Relax your breath and breathe in deeply.

Bring your attention to the center of your chest and imagine, as you inhale, that you are drawing into your body pure healing energy. Some people experience this as almost a liquid gold light, but you may need another ray in the color spectrum, so just let color come into you as it will. If you do not experience any color, trust this. Send loving energy into your breast through your hands. Exhale any negative thoughts that may arise. Offer gratitude for this opportunity to invite healing into yourself.

Sometimes, when we're too busy to pause and listen to the voice inside that tells us what we need, our bodies will do something that we cannot ignore, and it will get our attention.

Castor Oil Pack

Another effective compress, if you don't have access to gingerroot, is made with castor oil. This is an old Edgar Cayce treatment. Rub castor oil, preferably organic, over the area of your breast and cover this with a piece of either cotton or wool flannel. Place a hot-water bottle on top of the flannel and relax into this for twenty minutes.

Alby Poultice

Alby is a whitish powder made from clay and taro root, sometimes with ginger also, found in the Japanese section of a market. Mix 2 table-spoons with enough hot water to make a thick paste. You definitely do not want this to be runny. Apply the paste directly to the skin over the affected area of your breast. You can cover it with a piece of plastic wrap and place a hot-water bottle on top. Lie down and relax for twenty min-utes. You can follow the guided visualization in the ginger compress sec-tion if you like.

NURTURE YOURSELF—TIME OUT FOR YOU

If doing a meditation or visualization is just not your cup of tea, try to make this a pleasant, mellow, noninteractive time set aside just for your-self, without the pressure of feeling as if you must be doing something. And if this busyness feeling arises during your twenty-minutes-twice-daily-for-a-week time that you have set aside to assist in your healing, then take a good long look at what is behind the feeling. Do you feel guilty about taking so much time out of your busy, hectic schedule to do something nourishing for yourself? How often do you really take time for *you*? It's time to start—refer to the stress reduction and self-nurturing suggestions found throughout the book.

Many women have used this combination of treatments from differ-ent modalities and have avoided surgery to remove a noncancerous breast lump. By taking natural progesterone—100 mg twice a day, or a dosage tailored to reflect the values of the hormonal analysis—applying ginger compresses, an alby poultice, or castor oil packs, also twice a day, and taking a homeopathic remedy, one can more often than not avoid the surgeon's blade.

RX SUMMARY FOR BENIGN BREAST CONDITIONS

1. Compounded phytogenic natural progesterone therapy

   - Dosage based on your hormonal analysis, or
   - Progesterone: 100 mg twice a day for twenty-one days of your cycle, beginning with the cessation of menstrual bleeding or day six, whichever comes first

In addition to phytogenic progesterone therapy you may want to consider augmentation with:

2. Homeopathic remedies, specific to your profile; consider

For Fibrocystic Breasts
   - Calcarea Carbonica
   - Carbo Animalis
   - Carcinosin
   - Conium
   - Phosphorus
   - Phytolacca
   - Silica

For Mastitis
   - Belladonna
   - Bryonia
   - Hepar Sulphur
   - Phellandrium
   - Phytolacca
   - Pulsatilla

For Breast Abscess
   - Carbo Animalis
   - Hepar Sulphur
   - Phytolacca
   - Silica

For Galactorrhea
- Calcarea Carbonica
- Pulsatilla

3. Compresses, applied for twenty minutes twice a day for seven to ten days
4. Whole-foods diet

- Low in sugar
- Low in carbohydrates
- Low in fat
- High in protein
- High in fiber
- Avoid commercially raised meats and dairy containing exogenous hormones.
- Avoid refined, processed foods.
- Avoid caffeine and alcohol.

5. Support your immune functioning and restore balance.

- Immune enhancing
    Colloidal silver: 1 teaspoon three times a day for two weeks, followed by a daily dose for six months
    Olive leaf extract: 500–1,000 mg every six hours, beginning at the first sign of immune dysfunction
    Maitaki, shiitake, and reishi mushrooms, as directed
    Hawaiian noni, as directed
- Vitamins and minerals

6. Self-nurturance and stress reduction
7. Acupuncture
8. Aromatherapy to soothe

A FINAL NOTE

It is important to seek a professional exam and diagnosis on any breast lump. In many instances there is a grace period between the moment you discover a lump and when it may become imperative to remove it, and not all breast lumps must be removed. If your physician advises you that this is the case, you have some options you may wish to consider. You can simply watch the lump for signs of shrinkage or enlargement, or you can try the suggested treatments and see if your particular breast lump responds to a noninvasive approach. If the lump does not vanish or begin to reduce in size within this grace period, you should reevaluate and reassess your condition professionally.

9

ENDOMETRIOSIS

It is not my intention to rewrite the information now available on endometriosis. In recent years, much research has explored each aspect of this painfully challenging condition, the cause of which has yet to be clearly understood. My intention in this chapter is to give you another perspective, especially if you have been recently diagnosed with endometriosis or have had surgical intervention and want to prevent recurrence, if possible.

What is endometriosis? Each month in the normal flow of menstruation, we shed the lining of the uterus, the endometrium. By definition, endometriosis is a condition in which those same endometrial cells grow outside the uterus. These cells are commonly found on the ovaries, the outer uterus, the posterior cul-de-sac, the bowel, the ligaments that secure the uterus in place, the uterosacral ligaments, the anterior fold between the bladder and the uterus, throughout the pelvis in the peritoneum and abdominal cavity, or in more remote areas, such as the lungs and stomach.

A woman came to me many years ago after having surgery to remove endometrial tissue from behind her knee. This is unusual, but demonstrates the possibility of how far from the uterus endometrial tissue has been found. These cells depend on ovarian function and continue to cycle outside the uterus as though they were still in utero, responding to hormonal fluctuations and the normal cycling signals specific to ovarian function. This causes scar tissue and adhesions to build wherever the endometrial tissue implants.

CATEGORIES OF ENDOMETRIOSIS

Endometriosis is categorized in four stages, based upon its location:

- Stage I: superficial endometriosis with filmy adhesions—minimal disease
- Stage II: superficial endometriosis, filmy adhesions—mild disease
- Stage III: superficial and deep endometriosis, filmy and dense adhesions—moderate disease
- Stage IV: superficial and deep endometriosis, dense adhesions—severe disease

COMMON SYMPTOMS OF ENDOMETRIOSIS

Although there are some women who do not experience any symptoms, the following list is of those reported by most women who suffer with endometriosis.

1. Pain—mostly lower abdominal and specific to the pelvic area. The pain continues to worsen over the years and is primarily experienced:

- One to two days before bleeding begins and into menstruation (dysmenorrhea)
- Midcycle with ovulation
- Intermittently without a discernible pattern
- During intercourse, upon deep penetration, the pain may be unbearably piercing and agonizing (dyspareunia).
- In the bladder area and above the pubic bone
- On urination, sometimes showing blood in the urine
- With bowel movement

2. Depression
3. Irritability
4. Mood swings
5. Increased anxiety
6. Feelings of helplessness
7. Feeling fearful
8. Feelings of powerlessness

9. Feeling hopeless
10. Feelings of insecurity
11. Feeling worried
12. Heavy menstrual flow
13. Severe cramps during flow
14. Clotting during menses
15. Low backache before and/or during flow
16. Headaches before or with menstrual flow
17. Leg cramps
18. Bloating before and during menses
19. Prolonged menstrual flow, seven days of bleeding or longer
20. Regular cycle, though a shorter one of between twenty-one and twenty-six days from the beginning of one cycle to the beginning of the next
21. Continuous, uninterrupted, consistently regular cycle for five consecutive years
22. Repeated diagnosis of pelvic inflammatory disease (PID)
23. Difficulty with getting pregnant or inability to conceive

POSSIBLE CAUSES OF ENDOMETRIOSIS

Currently, there remains no proven cause of endometriosis. The most likely mode of transport of endometrial cells out of the uterus appears to be retrograde flow of menstrual bleeding into the fallopian tubes.

Other modes of transport may include:

- Lymphatic channels into other areas of the pelvis or other organs
- Blood vessels that carry endometrial cells to the lungs, skin, thighs, and extremities
- Surgery can spread or trap endometrial cells in the abdominal wall.

Some of the theorized but still unproven possible causes for endometriosis include:

- Elevated estrogen levels, especially as compared to the amount of progesterone
- Stressed immune system with increased susceptibility

- Exposure to external chemical toxins
- DES exposure: Some studies suggest that daughters of mothers who took diethylstilbestrol (DES) during their pregnancy for the prevention of miscarriage seem to have a higher incidence.

DIAGNOSING ENDOMETRIOSIS

Diagnosis of endometriosis is often missed or undetectable by pelvic exam and ultrasound. But if the endometrial implants are large enough, they can be seen on ultrasound. A blood test often used to screen for a tumor marker primarily for the ovaries, uterus, and fallopian tubes—CA125/CA125-II, a substance normally found in very low levels in the body—may be elevated if endometriosis is present but is not a definitive diagnosis. The risk of endometriosis developing into cancer is very low. But endometriosis can coexist with other pelvic disorders, such as uterine fibroids and ovarian cysts.

Laparoscopy, a surgical procedure using a scope to see inside the pelvic cavity, remains the primary method to obtain a definitive diagnosis. Recently, because women with pelvic pain and endometriosis measure elevated levels of CA125—the normal range by most labs is 35u/ml–45u/ml—there is consideration that a high CA125/CA125-II level in the presence of pelvic pain suggests a diagnosis of endometriosis.

If you decide, from all the research you have done, that you have endometriosis, it is probable that you do. And it could serve you well to discover your hormonal status via the salivary hormonal analysis to see if your progesterone is low.

NONSURGICAL, NATURAL TREATMENT OPTIONS FOR ENDOMETRIOSIS

PROGESTERONE THERAPY

Reread the list of common symptoms of endometriosis on pages 242–243 and think about the symptoms of insufficient progesterone and PMS.

See any similarities between the two? I am not a gynecological surgeon who treats thousands of women with endometriosis. Grateful as I am for all the skilled surgeons we have available to us, I prefer to prevent the need for surgery whenever it is possible. Is it possible that one of the underlying causes for endometriosis finds itself anchored in the imbalance of progesterone to estrogen? We understand that endometriosis requires ovarian function to develop. We see that when this function ceases, so do the symptoms that coexist with the condition. It is possible that without estrogen dominance, a term first used by John Lee, M.D., progesterone would not become suppressed or overpowered by elevated estrogen levels, and thereby become insufficient or completely deficient.

Emily's experience, age twenty-seven

I don't want to remain on birth control pills the rest of my life. Yet if I don't take the pill, the pain that starts just before my period is so intense, I can hardly breathe. Some months I would lie in bed, curled up in a ball, and cry myself in and out of sleep for days. I could hardly eat those days. Every time I ovulated, this overwhelming sense of fear and hopelessness would come over me. At least once I knew it was endometriosis, I didn't feel like I was out of my mind.

At twenty-seven, Emily had grown fearful of her body's own normal rhythms due to the severity of pain and the emotional side effects of the recurrent pain. As a professional single woman who was also going back to school to work on another degree, her life already had significant stress. Given the time constraints of working full-time and attending classes, her diet consisted of less whole foods and more sugars than she needed.

Believe me, I'm grateful for more manageable periods. But eventually I want to have a family. I don't know if that's really a possibility if I stay on the pill. Another thing I've noticed is that I seem to get sick more often than my friends. I'm young, for God's sake! I thought I was healthy. Does prolonged use of the pill compromise my immune system?

Emily wanted to do more than simply keep her endometriosis at bay by taking pills that shut off her ovulation. She felt scared the first month she went off the pill and began using a 10 percent progesterone cream twice a day from the time she stopped bleeding until the time her menses was to begin again. With significant effort, Emily modified her diet. She cut out refined products—the refined sugars, the pastas, the French baguettes. We discussed the possibility that her high stress level contributed to the endometriosis.

Determined to change her body's response, Emily agreed to try a natural approach, but she was not wild about using the cream. Even though she was working on the pace of her life, she wanted to swim before her first class and did not want to wait twenty minutes for the cream to be absorbed before going into the water. Capsules seemed easier and more realistic for Emily to maintain consistency and not miss a dose. Her prescription changed to 100 mg of progesterone taken orally every twelve hours for twenty-one days of the month. She also started taking a good multiple vitamin and mineral formula, antioxidants, and extra vitamin C. I added colloidal silver to her daily immune supportive regime, one-quarter of a teaspoon daily prophylactically for six months. If she felt a sore throat or cold coming on, she would increase the dosage to three or four times a day. And she agreed to make some changes in her life.

Six months later, Emily announced:

I quit my job and I'm going back to school full-time. I'm feeling better. And although I don't know if the endometriosis is gone, the pain seems to be. I want to stay on the progesterone through the school year, because I really do not want to risk having the kind of periods I had before I went on the pill. Then maybe I'll try going off it for a month or two and see what happens.

As with many women with a history of endometriosis, Emily responded well to the compounded phytogenic progesterone therapy, a change in her lifestyle to reduce stress, a good diet, and support to her immune system. As of the last time I saw her, she had not had another laparoscopy. She opted to continue this alternative, which supported her feeling of being proactive for herself, and helped her feel healthier and generally better than she did when she took birth control pills.

Emily is an example of the many women who chose to initiate significant changes in their lives. Altering one's lifestyle is not easy, especially for high-powered women in demanding professional positions who do not step into this kind of transformation without serious effort and commitment to themselves. When our self-image is validated by our professional life, how do we let it go and choose something more nurturing and less competitive . . . and healthier?

Erin's story, age forty-four

> I just can't go on like this any longer. My work is killing me. I can feel it in my bones. I was driving to my office when the pain gripped me so intensely I had to pull over. Talking to my secretary was a challenge. It almost felt like labor. I turned around and made it home, took a handful of ibuprofen, and went to bed with a hot-water bottle. I know I must change my life. Certainly no one else will do it for me. But I make decent money, have some freedom with my hours, and it's what I've done for a very long time.

After quite a bit of soul-searching, getting very real with herself, and choosing her health and well-being over her addiction to her professional image of herself, Erin decided to give herself time out to reevaluate her life and what she could do to support herself financially. She also went on a therapeutic regime similar to Emily's, 100 mg of progesterone twice a day for twenty-one days a month. As the executive in charge, she had always presented herself as the strong one, regardless of what was going on in her personal life or her body, so this was not an easy decision for her. What would people think of her for walking away? Some people supported her decision, while others were enraged by or unaccepting of it. Regardless, Erin knew that if she did not make a radical transformation in the pragmatic aspects of her life, her health would do it for her.

In addition to progesterone, vitamins, and a major lifestyle change, Erin also took homeopathic Nux Vomica 200C two times a day at midcycle through the first day of her next cycle. These supportive supplements helped relieve the edginess and emotional sense of hopelessness she felt with her experience of the endometriosis. Previously, she had felt trapped, as if there truly was no way out. She had acquiesced to the despair that she would have to bulldoze her way through life, and just keep working until it killed her.

> *I never meant to become a workaholic. But I was a single mom with few other resources that I could count on. But really, if I had contin- ued along that path of self-destruction, I would soon be no good to anyone. I'm learning a new way to be in this world, not feel like a victim of circumstance, and stop and say no when I need to. It's not been the easiest of transitions, but I am grateful I'm doing it.*

Erin had developed endometriosis quite a few years after she had given birth and plunged deeper and deeper into a profession that consumed most of her waking moments. Unlike Emily, her diet had been excellent for years and she had practiced yoga and meditation. Perhaps the com- bination of a high-stress position, little else in her life besides raising her daughter and work, and regular cycles, uninterrupted by any subsequent pregnancies, opened the door for the development of endometriosis. Sustaining a continued state of adrenal exhaustion for many years, Erin tended to be susceptible to getting the flu and was generally easily run down. But she kept on going, compensating for how she felt, driven by her commitment to her work. She continues to remain on the progester- one and supportive vitamins and has had twelve pain-free cycles as of this writing.

If you know you have endometriosis, or think that you do, there is hope for you to become symptom free and to heal not only the underly- ing cause but to prevent a recurrence of the condition.

STRESS REDUCTION AND LIFESTYLE REVISION

The type-A personality usually coexists with the condition of en- dometriosis. She is typically the go-getter of the group, ambitious, com- petitive, and she does whatever she has to do to get the job done, regardless of cost. And I do not mean monetary cost, because the cost is usually to herself. If you find yourself agreeing with any of this, please realize that part of a successful treatment requires you to change your life. And if you are a professional woman committed to long workweeks in a demanding job that pays you a good salary, a job that requires you to work fifty to sixty hours a week, and you still want to get pregnant, your life is out of balance.

I understand that you cannot work part-time and make partner, or cut back your hours and still get everything done. But trust me, it never all gets done. There is always something else that needs to be handled, some loose end that needs to be tied. And even if you leave work at a civilized hour, what about those piles of work you take home? You claim that it's necessary to show you're the equal of your male coworkers, so you won't be passed over for that next promotion. But do you really want that promotion and all the additional stress that comes with it? If you want to conceive, remain pregnant, and sustain a healthy body, maybe you don't. It's your choice. If you want to bring your work/ professional life into balance with your physical, mental, emotional, and spiritual well-being, it will require creative solutions. And that may mean you'll have to leave your work/job/profession for a healthier lifestyle. Or it may just mean you need to take a different perspective on how to do your job and to create a balance so you can also have a personal life.

As you uncover creative ways to simplify your daily life, consider what nurtures your being the most. What does your heart tell you to do? Can you hear beyond your mind's persistent nagging to that inner voice that speaks softly, and simply hear what you need to do right now, in this moment? A simple way that I have found to assist my mind is to write things down. This immediately takes it off my mind and frees me to be more present and in the moment.

Make a list of the things that nurture you, the things that you tell yourself you will find the time to do, just for you . . . someday. Here are a few ideas:

- Spend time in nature; go for a walk along a wooded pathway, a jungle or mountain trail, a path alongside a stream or on the beach.
- Find a peaceful place outdoors, whether in your yard, a nearby park, or a favorite space reasonably close by, and sit on that rock, on the ground, or on a bench. Now, do nothing but breathe in your surroundings.
- Take a class—in art, dance, theater, meditation, music, poetry, yoga, Dahn Hak, aerobics, crafts, puppet making, juggling, cooking, crea-

tive writing, linguistics, genealogy, geology, origami, archaeology, antiquing, music—in anything that makes you feel more connected to
yourself and more alive.

• Set aside a specific time each day to meditate or to just be with yourself in a positive, peaceful way. Let your inner self who longs for
magic arise and let her be born anew. Or simply be with yourself without judgment, without an agenda; accept the moment without the
need to make it into something else.

• Take time each day to acknowledge everything in your life for which
you are grateful. Make a small list of what you think is really important for you to have or accomplish at this time in your life. Now, offer
your thanks for each of these things as though you already have them.
Try to do this every day and allow yourself to feel it as real.

• Connect with your four-legged companions, play with them and love
them daily, and do something different with them or for them. Try
getting down on the floor and joining them in their playing. Allow
your inner playful beastie her expression.

• Pamper yourself. Get a facial, a pedicure, a massage, or something
you have never before done for yourself and your body, like taking a
mud bath. Use your imagination.

• Remind yourself of all the things you do that are creative, and if you
can't think of any, make a list of what you can realistically begin that
will inspire your sense of creativity. Even making a meal expresses
creativity. Now do the first thing on that list.

• Take an unscheduled afternoon off and go to a hot spring or spa, and
soak in the nourishing mineral baths.

• Take a tour of where you live and do it differently than you ever have
before—ride a bike, or walk with a friend and take turns saying out
loud, in a positive way, everything interesting that you each can notice.
Have fun with it and give yourself the gift of realizing another world
in your ordinary surroundings. Even if you live in a city where little of
nature can be found, see what surprises you can find when you choose
to see with your heart open and outside your ordinary perception.

Creative solutions to simplify our lives include any little time and energy
conservation device we can conjure up. I have an ongoing shopping list
in my computer, which I print out weekly; then I check off what is

needed rather than write a new list every time I need to go to the market. When I discover I have forgotten something, I add it to the master list, which contains, under each category and arranged in the order of the stores where I shop, everything I could ever need. This may sound like something trivial, but it saves me a surprising amount of time and mental energy. See if this helps you even a tiny bit. Here are the main categories I came up with. You may find others.

- Auto needs
- Bulk items
- Cards and presents
- Condiments
- Dairy foods (includes other refrigerated items where I shop)
- Dry goods
- Fresh fish
- Frozen items
- Fresh produce
- Household items
- Miscellaneous—I use this mostly for onetime items and delete them as I find them
- Office supplies
- Personal items
- Pet food and stuff
- Spices
- Teas

How do we maximize our time so that our waking hours serve us best? Discover if there is a particular period when you feel somewhat nonfunctional and tend to zone out in front of the TV or do something that could be simplified or even eliminated. Consider rearranging your schedule so you can sleep during this time instead. Cutting out whatever does not keep your energy level at its optimum or nurture your spirit will create the time elsewhere in your busy schedule to do things that will enhance your energy, vitality, and sense of well-being, such as meditation, reading something that inspires you, dancing, yoga, or a tai chi or chi gong class. It may also enable you to find your alone time, which you may have claimed does not exist.

If this nonfunctional time is in the middle of your workday and you do not work at home, your boss may not appreciate it. Perhaps you could find some way of incorporating personal energy work or body movement that does not create a problem at work. Or, if your nonfunctional time includes taking care of children, yours or someone else's, what can you do to nurture yourself as well? Can you add in the background music that feels good to you and soothes your spirit as well as the children's? Can you read aloud to the children books that can inspire you?

My mother always said: "Where there's a will, there's a way." This pops into my mind whenever I think I have run out of choices and I need to find a different way to see things. We always have a choice, even if it is to choose to change how we perceive something. If you see that you need to make changes in your life but feel clueless, just try doing something out of your norm to inspire you and evoke another point of view. You can choose to transform your life. We begin now, and now is a new moment.

REVOLUTIONIZE YOUR EATING

Does your hand reach for a candy bar when you need a meal? Do you slug down more coffee, or perhaps it's a diet soda, because you're so exhausted you can hardly keep your bleary eyes open, but you still have another couple of hours to go? Do you crave spicy foods, assuaged by alcohol? Or will just any stimulant do the trick? These are the very foods and drinks that pump you up and keep you going, that provide the illusion of energy. These are the very substances you need to avoid because they aggravate endometriosis. Consistent high caffeine intake during the day, countered by alcohol at night, stresses your adrenal glands, which in turn stresses your immune system.

What to eat? The supportive diet contains little sugar and none of the refined version. It is high in nutrients and vitamins, which occur naturally in the original source, not bleached or refined out and then chemically reintroduced, as in any enriched product. Energy requires fuel. Whole foods, preferably organic and devoid of added chemicals, pesticides, antibiotics, or exogenous hormones, equal fuel for the human body to achieve and sustain optimal health.

Commercially raised poultry and eggs contain hormones as well as other common additives. These exogenous hormones exacerbate and negatively feed your endometriosis, most often by increasing your estrogen levels. As excess estrogen seems to be part of the problem with endometriosis to begin with, the last thing you want to be doing is adding more. Organic meats and eggs do not contain added hormones or chemicals.

Refer to the dietary suggestions in the PMS section (page 60) as a guideline for the best way to nourish yourself and help your endometriosis. Use the following as a guideline of foods to avoid and foods to enjoy.

Foods to Avoid
Refined sugar
Bleached white flour breads, tortillas
Refined, enriched cereals and pastas
Any product containing refined sugars, bleached and enriched grains
Commercially raised poultry and eggs
Red meat
Alcohol
Coffee, black teas
Junk foods
Fast foods
Commercially canned products containing sugar and preservatives
Commercial salad dressings
All processed foods
Foods high in fats
Sodas, both regular and diet

Foods to Enjoy
Fresh, organic fruits and vegetables
Organic whole grains
Fresh fish, preferably deep-ocean
Fresh, organically fed, free-range poultry and eggs
Only organic dairy, and in limited amounts
Miso
Organic tofu, tempeh
Organic, caffeine-free teas
Stevia, as a substitute sweetener

Natural licorice, made from molasses, whole-wheat flour, licorice extract, anise seed oil

Organic popcorn, chips, and pretzels without sugar

Protein drinks, smoothies

A note on soy products regarding their estrogenic effects: You would need to consume extremely large quantities to appreciably increase your estrogen levels, but with endometriosis, you do not want to increase your estrogen. So if you digest soy products easily, enjoy them and eat a slight to moderate amount; you should not develop estrogen excess from your diet as long as you do not take in other exogenous estrogen sources.

HOMEOPATHY AND ENDOMETRIOSIS

The following is a brief synopsis of five primary remedies that help endometriosis. I'm including the personality-type picture of each remedy as well as the correlating symptoms, as a guide.

- *Apis* for the woman who develops cysts on the right ovary with her endometriosis, along with severe dysmenorrhea (excruciatingly painful periods). If she conceives, this woman is likely to spontaneously miscarry in the first trimester.
- *Lachesis* for the woman who experiences endometriosis more often affecting her left ovary along with severe dysmenorrhea, during which clothing, especially anything restrictive from the waist down, is unbearable. Her PMS symptoms are classically extreme with irritability, jealousy, paranoia, depression, intermittent angry outbursts, increased anxiety, and headaches. At times, she contemplates suicide.
- *Nux Vomica* for the woman whose endometriosis may involve her lower bowel, causing posterior pressure or the urge to pass stool with the onset of her dysmenorrhea. Her pain—uterine, lower back, and sometimes including bladder involvement—tends to be spastic and congested.
- *Pulsatilla* for the woman whose intense dysmenorrhea began at a young age, often from the beginning of her cycles at menarche. Her menses may be shorter than is usual for endometriosis, but they tend to be heavy and just as exquisitely painful, with the pain more pronounced in her lower left abdomen.

- *Sepia* for the woman whose symptoms are more severe on her left side, accompanied by an intense bearing-down sensation that feels as though her uterus will prolapse and fall out, particularly during her painful menstrual flow. Her PMS is marked with irritability to the point of yelling at loved ones, significant depression, and weeping despairingly. Sex becomes so painful (dyspareunia) that she may develop an aversion not only to sex but to being touched. Infertility is common, but if she does conceive after she has developed endometriosis, she is more likely to miscarry in the first trimester.

Another remedy that is not specific to endometriosis, but that I have found essential for women dealing with grief-provoking conditions, is *Ignatia*. Ignatia helps move the grief out of our cells and out of our bodies. Every woman I have ever met with a history of endometriosis has experienced much grief. Alternatively, if you do not see yourself in any of the above remedy profiles, a constitutional remedy tailored to your particular experience, including that of the endometriosis, may serve you best.

SUPPORT YOUR IMMUNE SYSTEM

In addition to finding the vitamin and mineral supplements you absorb and utilize well, extra B vitamins, antioxidants, and higher dosages of vitamin C remain important to augment and optimize your immune functioning. Please refer to the section on vitamins and minerals for PMS. For more details on specific immune support, refer to this section in Chapter 7 (page 211).

Also, as mentioned in Emily's and Erin's stories, colloidal silver is used to further support immune function.

In addition, it is also important to avoid adrenal exhaustion. To decrease stress to your adrenal glands, look at the pace of your life, and work on modifying your stress threshold and reducing it. You can test your adrenal function through a simple salivary sample taken at home and sent to a lab (see the list of labs in the Resources section) for testing. Make sure your adrenal glandular supplement is from an organically raised bovine source—that is, cows that are not given hormones or antibiotics. Taken for a period of three to six months, it could make a difference not only in boosting your energy but in repairing the damage.

Tailor your dosage to your deficiency as indicated by your salivary analysis, or based upon the severity of your symptoms.

Acupuncture is one of the best healing modalities to restore balance to an overstressed, less than optimally functioning immune system. Classic Chinese acupuncture does not talk about the immune system as a separate function, as in allopathic medicine. Taoists did not use that kind of terminology. Acupuncture does, however, address what is called Wei Qi, the qi energy or life force in the body that prevents external pathogens from entering, as defensive qi, and utilizes certain strong points for "clearing wind invasions." Recent studies reveal an increased production of white blood cells, the body's internal defense against infections, when specific acupuncture points have been stimulated. By tonifying the qi energy and blood (the concept of blood in Oriental medicine includes all substances transported by the blood), immunity becomes enhanced. This process assists in the elimination of toxins, thereby freeing the immune system to work more effectively without needing to battle with these excess toxins as well.

The Chinese herbal formula Cinnamon and Poria Formula (Gui Zhi Fu Ling Wan) is used for blood stagnation in the lower abdomen, fixed with masses, pain, and tension found in endometriosis. It reduces the masses caused by endometriosis, invigorates the blood, and repairs blood stagnation. There are many other Chinese herbs, specific to immune enhancement and support, that are best prescribed by a Chinese herbal practitioner who will tailor them to those areas where you need support.

RX SUMMARY FOR ENDOMETRIOSIS

1. Compounded phytogenic natural progesterone therapy:

   - Dosage based on your twenty-four-hour urine or salivary analysis
   - Progesterone: 100 mg twice a day for twenty-one days of your cycle, beginning with the cessation of menstrual bleeding or day six, whichever comes first

In addition to phytogenic progesterone therapy, you may want to consider augmentation with:

2. Lifestyle changes to lower daily stress, along with other stress reduction measures

- Make nurturing time for yourself, alone.
- Meditation
- Reevaluate your professional/work life.
- Exercise—yoga, tai chi, chi gong, dance
- Simplify daily life routines.
- Restructure your schedules.

3. Whole-foods diet

- Low in sugar
- Low in carbohydrates
- Low in fat
- High in protein
- High in fiber
- Avoid commercially raised meats and dairy
- Avoid refined, processed foods
- Avoid caffeine and alcohol

4. Homeopathic remedies, specific to your profile

- Apis
- Lachesis
- Nux Vomica
- Pulsatilla
- Sepia
- Ignatia

5. Adrenal glandulars to decrease adrenal stress and exhaustion

- Dosage based on your salivary analysis, or
- Dosage based on severity of symptoms correlated with the formula you choose

6. Evaluate your thyroid and treat appropriately.

7. Support your immune functioning.
8. Acupuncture
9. Herbal support; consider Cinnamon and Poria Formula
10. Vitamins and minerals

- B complex
- Calcium (1,200 mg)
- Magnesium (600 mg)
- Folic acid (100 mcg)
- Vitamin A (10,000 IU)
- Vitamin C (750–1,000 mg)
- Vitamin D (400 IU)
- Vitamin E (800 IU)
- Selenium (150 mcg)
- Zinc (45 mg)
- Essential fatty acids

SUPPORT SITES

Endometriosis Association, founded by Women for Women, *www.endometriosisassn.org/* or *www.endometriosis.org/*.

OVARIAN CYSTS

Olivia's experience, age twenty-five

> *My gynecologist put me on birth control pills because I kept devel-*
> *oping ovarian cysts. She called them "simple" cysts. But during some*
> *of my cycles the pain got so intense I spent two days in bed. That's*
> *when a cyst ruptured. It certainly did not feel simple, believe me. Can*
> *natural hormones help me stop developing cysts? And can natural*
> *hormones make my periods less painful, too?*

Olivia had a healthy diet and an active lifestyle full of sports and out-
door activities, minus at least two days each month.

As young women trying to avoid pregnancies, many of us have taken
birth control pills, which avert pregnancy by preventing ovulation. Some
practitioners believe that by turning off the ovarian function we prevent
ovarian cysts from forming. The ovaries cease to go through their normal rhythms of producing an egg and releasing it, and therefore will not
develop into a cyst if that tendency exists. Yet if a woman has this
propensity, within a short time of discontinuing the pill, her ovaries re-
vert back to the former pattern and again develop cysts. This is an example of what I call Band-Aid therapy. The pill may prevent a woman's
ovaries from making cysts due to the lack of ovulation. But it does not
really address the underlying problem of why her body makes cysts to
begin with.

If we inquire into the root cause on a physical level, we most often find that the woman is deficient in progesterone or that her progesterone pattern may be out of sync in relation to her estrogen. Either the progesterone levels are too low at the beginning of the cycle and never adequately reach the appropriate peak, or the progesterone levels rise too early in the cycle, peaking prematurely, resulting in the level dropping too low too soon. In this scenario, the estrogen levels may remain higher than the normal range throughout the entire cycle, or the testosterone levels may dominate, suppressing the manufacturing of sufficient progesterone.

Although I have not seen any study to substantiate my experience in working with more than one hundred women who have had ovarian cysts, as I've reflected on the stories they have shared with me, I recognized explicit and consistent emotional patterns that seem intertwined with occurrence of right-sided and left-sided ovarian cysts. Many women with cysts that recur on the right side have discovered that they have unresolved issues with the men in their lives—father, brother, lover, and/or husband. Whereas the women with left-sided cysts often seem to relate to the repeated sacrifice of the feminine, a pattern that so many of us repeat over and over as we try to compete in the previously male-dominated professional arena. We do what needs to be done, perhaps even more than is expected of us, regardless of where we are in our cycle, even if we are bleeding heavily and in the throes of gripping cramps. And we do this while juggling all the other tasks we are so adept at managing simultaneously. Sound familiar?

If we embrace and choose to live in the feminine paradigm, an entirely different way of stepping into this dance we call life, perhaps we can replace the race for success with an approach to taking action through our commitments to honor who we are with grace, gratitude, and trust. This commitment to action acknowledges that we bring the gift of our personal talents to a project, and rather than compete with one another, we can choose a cooperative relationship that negates no one, and that doesn't create a hierarchy for approval. This feminine paradigm requires us to surrender to what really is, with our eyes wide open to see this reality in its truth and not through the illusion of how we think it ought to be. It means letting go of old beliefs that perpetuate concepts such as that we are not good enough, we are too old to take on a new venture, we cannot do *it*, or there is not enough time and resources to meet the needs of everyone. Such old beliefs not only hold us back, they lock us into limiting our potential, which is our birthright. This disempowering practice no longer serves our physical, mental, emotional, and spiritual health. And through the wisdom of truly seeing what is, we can align ourselves with universal truth and can choose to take the right action from this resonance to truth and clarity.

So we want to resolve the underlying cause of this very common pelvic disorder, not just treat the symptom. If you have had more than one ovarian cyst diagnosed through either a pelvic ultrasound or a bimanual exam, at the hands of a skilled practitioner, and no other pathological cause has been identified, you may wish to evaluate your hormones. Either a twenty-four-hour urine collection, taken midcycle and again around day twenty, or the salivary analysis, collected throughout an entire cycle, will yield the patterns of your cycle. These tests clearly pinpoint the phases of the cycle during which your progesterone may need augmenting or supplementing.

Olivia discontinued her birth control pills and collected her saliva on the specified days throughout a normal cycle. This particular cycle revealed normal testosterone, estrogen, and DHEA levels. However, her progesterone levels danced all over the chart in the first half of her cycle, and then seemed to fade away around the time of ovulation on until her menses. Sick of taking pills every day, she opted to take her progesterone in drops under her tongue, beginning with a low dose of 35 mg. Olivia took her drops twice a day, increasing to 50 mg at midcycle, then to 100 mg for days twenty-two through twenty-seven, decreasing to 75 mg on day twenty-eight. She first noticed less pain with her next period, but with her second cycle off the pill, a small cyst developed on her right side.

Nonetheless, she continued to take the progesterone. In addition to progesterone therapy, she applied warm ginger compresses twice a day for ten days, beginning at midcycle. She also took homeopathic Apis Mel 200C twice a day. That incident became her final ovarian cyst to date. Her resolution took three cycles to complete. The fastest I have seen anyone eliminate an ovarian cyst has been within forty-eight hours, and the longest has been six months. Less than 1 percent of women with ovarian cysts did not respond to this treatment, and required surgical removal of the ovary and its cystic components.

Progesterone is also available in cream form over the counter, and in various sublingual forms—both drops and tablets. If you choose one of these products yourself, instead of getting a prescription from your practitioner, be sure the dosage in milligrams is stated on the label. For example, a 10 percent cream is equal to 100 mg per dosage. The better-quality progesterones are derived from wild yam or soy. The peanut sources have a greater incidence of allergic responses and do not seem to be absorbed quite as well.

If, like Olivia, you are currently experiencing a cystic enlargement of your ovary that is 5 cm or less in diameter, you may want to try one of, or a combination of, the following options in addition to progesterone therapy. Please be certain that your diagnosis suggests a cystic condition of your ovary rather than a tumor such as a dermoid, which is a non-malignant cystic tumor containing elements uncommon to the ovary, such as hair, teeth, or skin. It is reasonable to have a dermoid removed.

OTHER OVARIAN CYSTS

- *Chocolate cyst* is a cyst filled with a gelatinous chocolate-colored liquid. It represents debris from prolonged cyclic menstruation that was enclosed in the area surrounding the ovary at the site of endometriosis.
- *Mucoid cyst* is a cyst that develops from an excessive buildup of mucus that solidifies and encapsulates an area of the ovary.
- *Follicular cyst* is a cyst that arises from the follicle during the follicular phase of the menstrual cycle; it is the most common ovarian cyst.
- *Blood cyst* is a cyst that fills with blood; it can occur when a tiny blood vessel ruptures during ovulation.
- *Tubo-ovarian cyst* is an ovarian cyst that ruptures into the lumen of the tube.
- *Serous cyst* is a cyst filled with a thin, watery fluid.

YOUR NORMAL OVARY

Normally, a woman's ovaries are situated in the pelvic cavity on either side of the uterus. Each ovary consists of three primary sections. The follicular compartment enlarges to construct the follicle and normally ruptures midcycle to release the egg during ovulation. After ovulation, the

follicle collapses to create a hollow space and becomes the corpus luteum, the walls of which thicken and evolve into a compartment that
produces progesterone.

The ovarian stroma, the third section and a source of androgen hormones, secretes testosterone throughout a woman's life, even after the
ovary ceases to produce eggs. The stroma appears to be fibrous tissue in-
terconnecting the follicles.

NONSURGICAL TREATMENTS FOR OVARIAN CYSTS

NATURAL PROGESTERONE THERAPY

Many women have avoided the surgical removal of an ovarian cyst,
which often requires taking out the ovary (oophorectomy), with this
combination of treatments from different modalities. The compounded
phytogenic natural progesterone taken in an oral, sublingual, or transdermal method, either 100 mg twice a day, or a dosage tailored to reflect the
values of a hormonal analysis, restores hormonal balance. This, in combination with a ginger compress and a homeopathic remedy, more often
than not prevents the need for the surgeon's blade.

HOMEOPATHY FOR OVARIAN CYSTS

Olivia's right-sided ovarian cyst resolved with the continuation of the
progesterone and the application of a ginger compress for one week,
along with the homeopathic remedy. Ovarian cysts that develop on the
right side of the body usually respond quite nicely, and often quickly, to
a remedy called Apis Mel. The potency to take of Apis Mel is 200C, sublingually (under your tongue), two to four times a day for seven to ten
days. Also, unlike some other medicines, the remedy should not be taken
with food or liquids. Rather, it is best utilized when you have not eaten
for fifteen to twenty minutes before or after taking your remedy.

Homeopathic Remedies for Right-Sided Ovarian Cysts
- *Apis* for right-sided ovarian cysts, along with excruciatingly painful
  periods (severe dysmenorrhea)

- *Lycopodium* for right-sided ovarian cysts, and when the woman continues to sleep only on that side
- *Palladium* for right-sided ovarian cysts with pain that worsens from sudden movement or excitement. Unlike Lachesis and Naja, this remedy is for when the woman feels much better when lying on her left side.

Left-sided ovarian cysts have been trickier in my experience. In addition to taking natural progesterone, the remedy picture changes depending upon the nature of the cyst. It is best to evaluate the nature of the symptom and correlate this with the remedy or work with a good homeopathic physician from a constitutional approach, with the intent of restoring homeostasis throughout the entire being.

Homeopathic Remedies for Left-Sided Ovarian Cysts
- *Argentum Metallicum* for ovarian pain that arrives suddenly
- *Belladonna* for an ovarian cyst with sudden onset, and when the intensity of pain is exacerbated with any movement. The woman's skin over the pelvic region of the affected ovary may feel hot to the touch, marked with a sensation of much inflammation. There is significant tenderness with an intense throbbing or pulsing sensation. Bright red bleeding accompanies the rupture of a cyst.
- *Kali Bichromicum* for pain that radiates from the left-sided cyst, though not always
- *Lachesis* for when the woman is unable to lie on her left side—she will sleep only on her right. Her left ovary may pulsate with pain from the cyst.
- *Naja* is often difficult to distinguish from Lachesis, though it has a milder temperament. The woman's left-sided cyst will cause pain, and she cannot sleep on her left side.
- *Phosphorus* is for when the pain is worse when lying on the left side, the side of the woman's cyst or tumor.
- *Platinum* is for intense dysmenorrhea that is frequently accompanied by a bearing-down sensation associated with left-sided ovarian cysts.
- *Thuja* is for when uterine tumors develop as well as for left-sided ovarian cysts.
- *Ustilago:* Although I have never used this remedy, it is said by several homeopaths to treat left-sided swollen ovaries with a burning type of pain that radiates down into the woman's legs.

COMPRESSES AND POULTICES

Ginger Compress

Regardless of on which side the cyst has occurred, a hot compress will not only feel soothing, it will also help your body begin to break down the cellular components of the cyst and encourage reabsorption of the excess fluid. Refer to the directions in Chapter 8 (page 235) for how to make a hot ginger compress.

If you are visually oriented, picture a normal healthy ovary. See this as your own ovary while you place the compress directly on your skin over the site of your swollen ovary.

You can place a hot-water bottle on top to help maintain the temperature, or have a second cloth waiting in the tea to replace the first one when it cools down. A heating pad may seem more convenient, but we really don't know what happens to the electrical current of our bodies when we add an external source of electricity with things like heating pads and electric blankets. Many people believe that these things disrupt the naturally occurring magnetic field of the human body. Hot-water bottles are inexpensive and easy to deal with when we need to increase or sustain a warmer temperature in specific and relatively small areas.

Allow your mind to focus on your ovary. Go inside with your mind's inner vision, your inner knowing, and connect with your ovary. Does any particular image arise? Ask this inner knowing, the wisdom of your true self, if there is anything your ovary wishes to communicate to you.

Years ago a friend shared with me a quote from a medicine man who lived in the Taos, New Mexico, pueblo: "Worrying is praying for what you do not want." When we investigate and discern the truth or as close to it as we can get, the mind's need to know has been satisfied and we don't need to worry. Rather, we can focus on the appropriate action. This quote has stuck with me and instigated my own investigation into the power of negative prayer. As I understand the workings of the mind, where we focus our thought patterns, energy has no choice but to follow. And when we continually focus on what is wrong or what is not working, we are putting our attention into the negative, hence, negative prayer.

Back to you in your resting place, visualizing your ovary. Let any form of connection and communication reveal itself. Try not to control it or even grasp a meaning just yet. Just breathe into your ovary. Send loving energy into your lower abdomen. One way to do this, but not the only way, is to place your hands on your pelvis, just inside your pelvic bone, fingertips facing one another, thumbs about an inch or two below your navel, depending on the length of your torso. The warm ginger compress rests below your palm on the side requiring attention.

Bring your attention to the center of your chest and imagine, as you inhale, that you are drawing into your body pure healing energy. Exhale any negative thoughts that may arise. Offer gratitude for this opportunity to invite healing into yourself.

Sometimes when we're too busy to pause and listen to the voice inside, our body will do something that we cannot ignore in order to get our attention. I can speak from personal experience because during this past year I developed cysts in my left ovary, more than once. For me, I discovered that I had to step away from operating out of an old paradigm, which was definitely to *put work first, no matter what it takes, and keep pumping hard to get the job done.*

Part of my own healing has come through learning my own rhythm with work, connecting with others, moving my body and learning to pay attention to what is really going on in each moment—to see things as they actually are rather than how I think I might want them to be. Bringing into balance the communication of body and mind through moving the body, engaging the mind, balancing my hormones, and working with my energy has deeply affected how I relate to myself and everything else.

Castor Oil Pack and Alby Poultice
Refer to the directions in Chapter 8 (page 237).

RX SUMMARY FOR OVARIAN CYSTS

1. Compounded phytogenic natural progesterone therapy

   - Dosage based on your twenty-four-hour urine or salivary analysis, or
   - Progesterone: 100 mg twice a day for twenty-one days of your cycle, beginning with the cessation of menstrual bleeding or day six, whichever comes first

In addition to phytogenic hormone therapy, you may want to consider augmentation with:

2. Whole-foods diet
3. Homeopathic remedies, specific to your profile and the cyst's location

For right-sided ovarian cysts consider:
- Apis
- Lycopodium
- Palladium

For left-sided ovarian cysts consider:
- Argentum Metallicum
- Belladonna
- Kali Bichromicum
- Lachesis
- Naja
- Phosphorus
- Platinum
- Thuja
- Ustilago

4. Compresses and poultices
5. Balanced vitamins and minerals
6. Acupuncture
7. Chinese herbs: Cinnamon and Poria Formula, three tablets three times a day, or the dosage recommended by your practitioner
8. Stress reduction measures:

- Make nurturing time for yourself, alone.
- Meditation

9. Support your immune system.
10. Exercise—yoga, tai chi, chi gong, dance

11

UTERINE FIBROIDS

YOUR NORMAL WOMB, THE UTERUS

Within a woman's womb meets the energy of heaven and earth. It is our midpoint; it is from where we draw on the abundance of resources from above, heaven, and the grounded energy from below, the earth. We have the ability to take both deeply into our bodies, into our being. We may use these resources to bring creativity to anything, whether it is to prepare a meal, make the home inviting to all who enter, make a baby, complete an artistic endeavor or business project. Anything we can imagine holds a creative potential, and it is through our womb that we access power from heaven and earth if we choose to.

Physically, our womb, the uterus, is a pear-shaped muscular organ lined by a mucous membrane, the endometrium, that is held in the mid-pelvis by two broad ligaments. Consisting of three sections, the largest is the round, expanded portion, the body, which constricts into the central area, the isthmus. Situated above the fallopian tubes, the roundest and uppermost aspect is the fundus. The lowest portion, the cervix, within reach through the vagina, includes a portal to the inside of the uterus through the cervical os. The os allows sperm entry to penetrate an egg in conception and provides an exit for the shedding of the endometrial lining each month as well as birth, miscarriage, or abortion. A uterine fibroid that develops in the inner layer near the endometrium can also abort in a similar manner.

As a flexible structure, the womb may rest in varied positions: *anteverted*, bending slightly forward, toward the pubic bone; *anteflexed*, bending completely forward; *retroverted*, leaning backward; and *retroflexed*, bending completely backward. Within these four angles, the uterus rests either in the middle of the pelvis or may incline toward either the right or left side. Displacement toward either side may be caused by growths, such as an ovarian cyst, or by the weight of fibroids, or due to no apparent anomaly.

Fran's story, age thirty-six

Fran developed uterine fibroids long before any menopausal symptoms began. As we suspected, her progesterone levels were quite low throughout her entire cycle. When she did not notice any change while taking her progesterone orally, I switched her approach to the transdermal route, 100 mg of progesterone in a cream form. She targeted her primary site of application directly over the fibroids. The fibroids did not get larger, but they did not shrink, either.

> I feel really frustrated. These lumps in my belly make me look perpetually pregnant and way worse when I eat a normal-size meal. I constantly have to pee from the pressure. And sex is just awkward. Bob bumps up against this hard lump inside of me. It's gross! I certainly lose the mood, let me tell you . . . Am I looking at surgery at this stage?

For the next six months, Fran took progesterone in vaginal suppositories five days a week, but not during her bleeding time. I increased her dosage to 400 mg. The fibroids became smaller. She noticed that when she forgot to take a suppository, her breasts became rather tender.

> Whenever I forget my progesterone, my breasts get so sore. Bob tried to give me a hug one day. He wanted to tell me he still loved me even though we hadn't made love in months, and I shrieked at the pressure of his touch. It hurt too much to hug him. Needless to say, I became very consistent with the treatment. And look, my belly has gone down.

Fran opened her sarong skirt and proudly displayed her more-normal-to-her abdomen. And the exam and ultrasound agreed; the fibroids were smaller.

Fiona's story, age fifty-one

When Fiona first came to see me, she had been offered a hysterectomy as her only option to treat her fibroids. She bled so profusely each month that she fainted from anemia and the hemorrhaging. Although she had no desire to become pregnant at fifty-one, she preferred to keep her uterus. Her most recent menses sent her to the emergency room hemorrhaging, and she had another D&C. Her endometrial biopsy was negative for malignancy.

I feel so weak from this bleeding. In two days I saturated twenty-four of the thick OB pads and my clothes. The bleeding and hard cramping make me feel sick with waves of nausea and heart palpitations, and I feel very stressed. My breasts become quite tender while all this is happening.

The initial focus for Fiona was to get the heavy bleeding under control, which was accomplished in three days by taking 200C of Aconite four times a day and 100 mg of natural progesterone four times a day initially and then decreasing to twice a day. This treatment held through one cycle until her next menses arrived, flooding with profuse bright red bleeding and the passing of many large clots. Twenty minutes after I gave her a dose of 1M of Belladonna, her bleeding stopped. She resumed taking her progesterone and kept the 1M of Belladonna on hand for emergencies.

Over the next two years Fiona would occasionally require a dose of Belladonna, though a lower dose of 30C sufficed. Her fibroids and bleeding became less disturbing as her cycle began to appear more like a pinkish mucous discharge. I added 0.625 mg of biestrogen and 2 mg of testosterone in separate drops to be taken sublingually because her energy remained quite low.

I feel stronger when I take the estrogen now, more energetic.

Four years later Fiona ceased to have periods, and before she became postmenopausal, her fibroids had resolved completely. The hemorrhaging and fears of surgery previously plummeted her into despair and deeper fears of dying. She continued to take her progesterone in a 10 percent cream and 1.25 mg of biestrogen in sublingual drops. She looked like a radiant, vibrant new woman at her last visit, six years after we first met.

Frederica's story, age fifty-one

My doctor put me on Triphasil, a birth control pill. He also offered me a hysterectomy because my periods have become so heavy. I must get up during the night to change these big heavy-duty OB pads every twenty minutes on the heaviest days, and every hour and a half to three hours on my lighter days. I feel so exhausted and depleted that I barely function. I feel like I'm dying. The birth control pills made no difference, so I stopped taking them. Last month I had to go to the emergency room because I hemorrhaged. Is a hysterectomy my only choice?

Frederica shook with weariness and fear as she shared her monthly experiences. She could not endure much more of this either physically or emotionally. Although she had been diagnosed with uterine fibroids eight years earlier, it was not until she had turned fifty-one that they became problematic. I started her on 100 mg of progesterone with 5 mg of testosterone orally, twice a day, with the same amount of hormones in a transdermal cream to apply directly on her lower pelvic area, the site of a substantial fibroid. She also began taking a time-release iron capsule with vitamin C, 30C of homeopathic Aconite four times a day, and the herb Shepherd's Purse in a tea. She also applied warm ginger compresses, which seemed soothing to her.

Frederica could not take the progesterone in vaginal suppositories because of the heavy bleeding, which would negate any potential absorption and actually expel the suppository before it could dissolve. Her next menses, early yet again, seemed less heavy and without clotting. She then had one normal cycle before the heavy bleeding pattern resumed. Her next formula contained a higher dose of testosterone, 10 mg, and the same progesterone. In addition to the other remedies, she began taking Ume concentrate four times a day. Made from the Japanese umeboshi plum, the plum extract decreases the acidity in the gut and enhances the absorption potential of other ingested nutrients as it alkalinizes the digestive tract.

Frederica's cycles became irregular as she continued to approach menopause. I removed the testosterone from her oral prescription and had her use it separately in a 5 mg per gram cream, applied directly to the fibroid via her pelvic and labial regions. She also began taking 200C of Sabina (had this not been effective, the next remedy would have been Ustilago). Her menses became much more normal after increasing her progesterone to 100 mg four times a day for three months.

> It's amazing. My bleeding is much lighter, hardly any clotting. I feel better—I'm sleeping again with no fatigue during the day. And look, my nails are growing and getting hard again, my hair is coming in thicker. All this changed within a month of the new prescription.

OTHER TREATMENT OPTIONS THAT HELP SHRINK FIBROIDS

NATURAL PROGESTERONE AND TESTOSTERONE THERAPY

Some women will benefit by augmenting the progesterone with testosterone if they are deficient. Sometimes progesterone alone can reduce the size of uterine fibroids, but frequently testosterone facilitates a significant change.

The first uterine fibroid I discovered on a bimanual exam, confirmed by ultrasound, was in 1986. This woman was not yet into the perimenopausal phase, but she felt some vague pelvic discomfort. Fortunately, her fibroid was discovered early in its development, when it was the size of a large walnut. With natural progesterone, alby poultices, and acupuncture, it resolved completely in two months.

HOMEOPATHY

- *Aurum* for fibroids accompanied by grief
- *Aconite* is useful for uterine hemorrhage.
- *Belladonna* for sudden onset of bright red bleeding from uterine fibroids, with intense pain exacerbated by any movement. The skin

over the pelvic region may feel hot to the touch, and there is significant tenderness with an intense throbbing or pulsing sensation.

- *Calcarea Carbonica* for significant hemorrhage with fibroids
- *Conium* for a slow progression with tumors common in the uterus and ovaries
- *Ferrum* for flushes with excessive bleeding from fibroids
- *Helonias* primarily focuses on female hormonal issues and uterine dysfunctions. The Helonias woman has an awareness of her womb all the time, feeling any change of its position as she moves.
- *Kali Bromatum* for uterine fibroids more on the right side
- *Kali Carbonicum* for uterine fibroids with possible bleeding between menses or absent cycles
- *Kali Ferrocyanatum* for profuse, painless hemorrhaging, taking the woman into radical anemia, with her uterine fibroids
- *Phosphorus* is another good remedy for uterine fibroids.
- *Sabina* for dysmenorrhea as well as other uterine disorders, and for bleeding between menses with a gushing of bright red blood and clots, worse from uterine fibroids
- *Tarentula Hispanica* for bleeding between normal cycles and for a burning sensation in the uterus
- *Thuja* for uterine tumors with a tendency toward fibroids on the left side
- *Ustilago* for fibroids with a burning type of pain that may radiate down into the legs

GINGER COMPRESSES, CASTOR OIL PACKS, ALBY POULTICES

Refer to the directions in Chapter 8 (pages 235 and 237).

Do not forget to take time out to be nurturing to yourself. The ginger compresses, castor oil packs, or alby poultices can be beneficial when placed directly over the center of the lower abdomen. If you can feel your fibroid through the surface of your lower abdomen, it may feel as hard as a billiard ball, but your ability to feel it depends on where in your uterus the fibroid is located. Fibroids can grow on the outside of the uterine wall, in between the layers of the uterine muscle, or in the inner layers of the uterus. The easiest fibroids for a woman to actually palpate on herself are those that grow on the outside layer of the uterus.

The earlier fibroids are diagnosed, the easier they are to resolve, or at least you can slow the growth rate and reduce the size. Fibroids grow at an undefined pace, dependent on hormonal and genetic influencing factors. A 2 cm fibroid responds more quickly to nonsurgical intervention than does a fibroid the size of a football.

WOMB MEDITATION

Sit on the floor in a comfortable cross-legged position. If you are unable to sit on the floor, sit in a firm chair with your legs slightly open. Gently rest your hands, palms facing upward, on your knees. Feel your entire body free of any self-judgments and self-doubts; accept yourself as you are at this very moment. Connect with your body, feel the pulse of your external genitalia touching the ground or your seat's surface.

Envision the expansiveness of the universe around you out into the cosmos, and the infinite existence of energy within this vastness. Focus on the top of your head as a receptor for pure energy from this incalculable resource. Inhale slowly, deeply, and feel the energy pour into you through the top of your head. Imagine this energy in the form of an element, such as light—like sunlight or in a specific color—or as a pristine waterfall. Trust how the energy presents itself to you, as what you need in this moment. Exhale the toxins, fears, and anything that does not work for you in your life. Let them go, even if only for this moment.

Feel this energy move downward through the midline of your body, nourishing each of your centers, your primary chakras, and replenishing you. We have channels of energy circuits throughout the body, all of which are interconnected. Imagine these channels to be open, the energy flowing unobstructed, balanced with love, forgiveness, compassion, and trust. Inhale as you draw in this expansive energy from heaven through the top of your head down through your centers and into your womb, contact the earth by breathing the earth energy in through your vagina, or yoni, as some women prefer, and imagine the grounded strength of the earth enter and fill your womb. Exhale the impurities. Feel your inhalation take these infinite resources directly to your womb and say thank you to the healing coming into you. Exhale whatever does not belong to you now, that may be stored in your womb, and tell it, "You can go now." Heaven and earth meet as we open these channels, breathing in resources from both.

Take a few moments to experience the visceral level of this energy. Feel renewed aliveness in your pelvis. You may want to place your hands over your lower abdomen and send love into your womb, gently, without any expectations, but simple love for what is. Contemplate things about yourself and your life for which you feel gratitude. Offer that gratitude to the Universe/the Creator/God/Goddess/Spirit of your personal spiritual path. Extend gratitude for this opportunity to be present with yourself, with your womb, to experience this merging of heaven and earth inside you.

RX SUMMARY FOR UTERINE FIBROIDS

1. Compounded phytogenic natural progesterone and testosterone therapy, twice a day:

   - Dosage based on your twenty-four-hour urine or salivary analysis, or
   - Progesterone: 100 mg twice daily for twenty-one days of your cycle, beginning with the cessation of menstrual bleeding or day six, whichever comes first
   - Testosterone: 5–10 mg, twice daily

In addition to phytogenic hormone therapy, you may want to consider augmentation with:

2. Whole-foods diet, with particular attention to:

   - Fresh fish and/or organic, free-range poultry
   - Avoid commercially raised meats and dairy (which contain exogenous hormones).
   - Avoid refined, processed foods.
   - Decrease caffeine and alcohol.

3. Homeopathic remedies, specific to your profile:

   - Aconite
   - Aurum

- Belladonna
- Calcarea Carbonica
- Conium
- Ferrum
- Helonias
- Kali Bromatum
- Kali Carbonicum
- Kali Ferrocyanatum
- Phosphorus
- Sabina
- Silica
- Tarentula Hispanica
- Thuja
- Ustilago

4. Vitamins, minerals, and antioxidants—find a good balanced formula that you can absorb easily.
5. Chinese herbs—Cinnamon and Poria Formula three times a day
6. Compresses and poultices
7. Stress reduction measures:

   - Make nurturing time for yourself, alone.
   - Womb meditation

8. Acupuncture
9. Support your immune system.
10. Exercise—yoga, chi gong, tai chi, dance, swim, walk

EPILOGUE: PERHAPS IT'S TIME TO STOP POURING TEA FOR EVERYONE

But now that I am in love
with a place that doesn't care
how I look and if I am happy,
happy is how I look and that's all . . .
—Fleur Adcock, "Weathering"

That place we want to love is within us, devoid of the expectations of who we think we were programmed to become, of how we think we ought to be. And we can stop trying to pretend that we must do life the way a culture dictates it and discover our own way, one of the beauties of embracing our authentic selves. When we welcome our own evolution, including the aging process, we step into grace.

The years work their weathering, but we can soften the lines of time with hormonal balancing. Yet the real softening occurs someplace deep within the psyche when we stop trying to pour tea for everyone, when we stop trying to be nice all the time and instead find the greater peace in being real with who we are in our essence. This is self-compassion. If we are to be compassionate with others, we must learn to begin with ourselves. This requires discernment without judgmental behavior, and forgiveness of everything that triggers a reaction within us. We can discover how to say no, simply and without feeling guilty. We do not need to await a cancer diagnosis or catastrophic event to step into *now* as the most important moment. And, like establishing any new pattern, it takes practice. If we truly desire to live in a world of peace, we must choose to create it within ourselves first.

Know thyself. We've heard this expression throughout our lives. The process and changes we go through during life's transitions challenge this beyond our wildest dreams. Yet by revealing ourselves to one another, we reveal self to self. Contained within this raw truth, we create a gateway to freedom, to awakening. Our journeys take us here. And it is these journeys that matter, not just the goal. Good journey to you.

PART FOUR

RESOURCES

DIRECTORY

COMPOUNDING PHARMACIES

International Academy of Compounding Pharmacists, IACP: IACP is a non-profit organization that provides a compounding referral service.

P.O. Box 1365; Sugar Land, TX 77487
Tel: 800-927-4227
Website: *www.iacprx.org*
E-mail: *iacpinfo@iacprx.org*
Executive director: L. D. King

Professional Compounding Centers of America, PCCA: More than three thousand members throughout the United States, Canada, Australia, and New Zealand. Customer Service identifies compounding pharmacists in your area for prescribing practitioners and women who call in for referrals.

9901 South Wilcrest Drive; Houston, TX 77099
Tel: 800-331-2498
Fax: 800-874-5760
Website: *www.pccarx.com*
E-mail: *deannat@pccarx.com*

Women's International Pharmacy, WIP: Prepares custom medications to prescribing practitioner's order. They carry DHEA, pregnenolone, micronized progesterone, all three estrogens, testosterone, natural thyroid, and thousands of other prescription medications. They also carry an olive leaf extract formula called Olivirex. Hormone replacement formulas are their specialty.

P.O. Box 6468; Madison, WI 53716
Tel: 800-279-5708
13925 W. Meeker Boulevard, #13
Sun City West, AZ 85375
Website: *www.womensinternational.com*
Pharmacist: Wallace L. Simmons

LABORATORIES

Aeron Lifecycles: Offers saliva hormone testing services, many on an over-the-counter basis, sex steroids, corticosteroids, melatonin.
   1933 Davis Street, Suite 310; San Leandro, CA 94577
   Tel: 800-631-7900
   Fax: 510-729-0383
   Website: *www.aeron.com*
   E-mail: *aeron@aeron.com*

Diagnos-Techs, Inc.: Provides extensive salivary hormonal, thyroid, and adrenal testing as well as bone marker, intestinal pathogen/health panels, and melatonin biorhythms. They require an order from your practitioner, to whom they send results.
   P.O. Box 58948; Seattle, WA 98138-1948
   Tel: 800-878-3787
   Fax: 425-251-0637
   Website: *www.diagnostechs.com*

Doctor's Data, Inc. & Reference Laboratory: Offers many tests including blood, urine, and hair analysis.
   P.O. Box 111; West Chicago, IL 60185
   Tel: 800-323-2784 (USA and Canada) 630-377-8139 (elsewhere)
   Fax: 630-587-7860
   Website: *www.doctorsdata.com*
   E-mail: *inquiries@doctorsdata.com*

Great Smokies Diagnostic Laboratory: Provides many tests, including salivary hormonal analysis, vitamin and hair analysis, and bone marker.
   63 Zillicoa Street; Asheville, NC 28806
   Tel: 800-522-4762
   Website: *www.gsdl.com*

Rhein Consulting Laboratories: Provides hormonal testing using twenty-four-hour urine method for measuring estrogens, testosterone, DHEA, the metabolite of progesterone, corticosteroids, and adrenal stress, and they will soon be offering alpha hydroxi to screen for breast cancer. They require an order from your practitioner, to whom they send results.

4475 SW Scholls Ferry Rd., Suite 101; Portland, OR 97225

Tel: 503-292-1988

Fax: 503-292-2012

Website: *www.rheinlabs.com*

E-mail: *fjnordt@rheinlabs.com*

Director: Frank Nordt, Ph.D.

OTHER NATURAL PRODUCTS

United States Sources

Allergy Research Group: It is their purpose to improve the quality of people's lives through scientifically based innovation, purity of ingredients, education, and outstanding service. They are an excellent source of organic adrenal glandulars and bovine thyroid.

30806 Santana Street; Hayward, CA 94544

Tel: 800-545-9960

TTY: 800-676-5274

Worldwide: 510-487-8526

Fax: 800-688-7426 or 510-487-8682

Website: *www.allergyresearchgroup.com*

E-mail: *info@allergyresearchgroup.com*

Amazon Herb Company: Specializes in rain forest bioenergetics and is committed to ensuring the integrity of product quality while supporting ecological integrity of the rain forest and its inhabitants.

1002 Jupiter Park Lane; Jupiter, FL 33458

Tel: 800-835-0850

Fax: 561-575-7935

Website: *www.rainforestbio.com*

E-mail: *orders@amazonherb.com*

ArxC, Alternative Medicine Connection: Provides the connection for ordering on-line many high-quality nutritional resources, such as Alacer Corp., Ecological Formulas, and Nutricology.

Website: *www.arcx.com*

E-mail: *abrecher@arxc.com*

Beyond a Century: Carries performance nutritional products, amino acid mixtures, antioxidant formulas, athletic and weight-loss formulas, meal replacements, sterol creams, skin and hair products.

HC 76, Box 200; Greenville, ME 04441

Tel: 800-777-1324

Fax: 207-695-2492

Website: *www.beyond-a-century.com*

E-mail: *nutrition@beyond-a-century.com*

Bio-Botanical Research, Inc.: Synergistic combinations of botanicals have been chosen from healing traditions worldwide for their specialized formulations. The broad-spectrum activity of these botanicals has been verified by laboratory testing and clinical usage.

2110 Dolphin Drive; Aptos, CA 95003

Tel: 800-775-4140

Fax: 831-688-5818

Website: *www.biobotanicalresearch.com*

E-mail: *info@biobotanicalresearch.com*

Medical herbalist: Rachel Fresco Salanda, L.Ac.

Biomed Comm, Inc.: Produces a variety of dietary supplement products based on nanomolar-strength and homeopathic cell-signaling factors (cytokines), including growth hormone, IGF-1, TGF-beta3.

2 Nickerson Street, Suite 102; Seattle, WA 98109

Tel: 888-637-3516 or 206-284-3433

Fax: 206-284-6585

Website: *www.biomedcomm.com*

E-mail: *info@biomedcomm.com*

BIOS Biochemicals: Sells powdered amino acids, including L-tryptophan, for pet food and veterinary use in quantities from 50 grams to multiple kilos. Their tryptophan is USP (pharmaceutical) grade, greater than 99.9 percent pure, and is "free of pyrogen and EBT."

P.O. Box 27848; Tempe, AZ 85285-7848
Tel: 800-404-8185 or 480-858-0502
Fax: 480-858-0547
Website: *www.biochemicals.com*
E-mail: *bios@biochemicals.com*

Ecological Formulas: An innovative developer of specialty nutritional products.
1061-B Sharly Circle; Concord, CA 94518
Tel: 800-888-4585
Fax: 925-827-2636
Website: *www.arxc.com/formulas/ecoform.htm*

Eden Foods, Inc.: Has offered the highest-quality, purest, traditionally prepared, whole foods for more than thirty years. They have built a dedicated network of family farmers who grow their food, and they can trace any Eden organic food to the field where it was grown and the seed it was grown from.
701 Tecumseh Road; Clinton, MI 49236
Tel: 888-441-3336 or 888-424-3336
Website: *www.edenfoods.com/*
E-mail: *info@edenfoods.com*

Enzyme Process International: Specializes in nutritional food concentrates and nucleic acid, liquezyme specific combination formulas, homeopathics, herbs, and vitamins.
Dept. CN, 2035 East Cedar Street; Tempe, AZ 85281
Tel: 800-521-8669 or 480-731-9290
Website: *www.enzymeprocess.com*
E-mail: *info@enzymeprocess.com*

Golden Flower Chinese Herbs: Provides practitioners with traditional and innovative herbal formulas that are easy to take and address symptom patterns seen in modern clinical practice. These high-quality products are without the impurities or questionable ingredients found in some of the patent formulas available.
P.O. Box 781; Placitas, NM 87043
Tel: 800-729-8509 or 505-837-2040
Fax: 866-298-7541 or 505-837-2052
Website: *www.gfcherbs.com/*
E-mail: *gfch@aol.com*

The Green Turtle Bay Vitamin Co., Inc.: Includes Sunnie (includes St. John's wort and Betaine TMG) as well as other fine vitamin formulas, and ships worldwide.

    56 High Street; Summit, NJ 07901
    Tel: 800-887-8535 or 908-277-2240
    Fax: 908-273-9116
    Website: *www.energywave.com*
    E-mail: *mail@EnergyWave.com*

Hahnemann's Laboratories: An excellent resource for quality homeopathic remedies.

    1940 Fourth Street; San Rafael, CA 94901
    Tel: 888-4-ARNICA or 888-427-6422
    Fax: 415-451-6981
    Website: *www.hahnemannlabs.com/*
    Pharmacist: Michael Quinn

Heel, Inc.: Provides quality combination homeopathic remedies based on a specific German formulary.

    11600 Cochiti Road SE; Albuquerque, NM 87123-3376
    Tel: 800-621-7644 or 505-293-3843
    Fax: 505-275-1672
    Website: *www.heelbhi.com*
    E-mail: *info@heelbhi.com*

Holliday's Herbals: It is their intention to bring healing through pure plant medicine to those who need it, providing the simplicity of nature in their products. Free catalog.

    P.O. Box 2878; Santa Fe, NM 87504
    Tel: 800-755-0182 or 505-988-3003

KAL Supplements: A distributor of quality nutritional supplements to health food stores—if they can't direct you to a local store, they will fill your order directly.

    6415 De Soto Avenue; Woodland Hills, CA 91365
    Tel: 800-755-4525
    Website: *www.thebetterhealthstore.com* or *www.vitaminlife.com*
    Order on-line: *www.totaldiscountvitamin.com/merchant/kal/htm*

The KEY Company: Dedicated to helping people achieve happy and healthy lives through education and prevention. They provide quality herbal, nutritional, and hard-to-find products.

    1313 West Essex Avenue or P.O. Box 220370; St. Louis, MO 63122

    Tel: 800-325-9592 or 314-965-6699

    Fax: 800-455-0306 or 314-965-7629

    Website: *www.thekeycompany.com*

    E-mail: *info@thekeycompany.com*

Life Enhancement Products, Inc.: A source for many specialty cognitive nutrition supplements, some of which are formulated by Ward Dean, M.D., and Durk Pearson and Sandy Shaw.

    P.O. Box 751390; Petaluma, CA 94975

    Tel: 800-543-3873 or 707-762-6144

    Fax: 707-769-8016

    Website: *www.life-enhancement.com*

    E-mail: *info@life-enhancement.com*

LifeLink: Sells DHEA, 5-hydroxytryptophan, and pregnenolone. They also carry high-potency extracts. Free catalog.

    750 Farroll Road; Grover Beach, CA 93433

    Tel: 888-433-5266 or 805-473-1389

    Fax: 805-473-2803

    Website: *www.lifelinknet.com*

    E-mail: *lifelinknet.com*

Longevity Formulas: The best resource for quality, consistently effective colloidal silver. They maintain a line of other nutritionals, such as Hawaiian Noni.

    Las Vegas, NV 89102

    Tel: 800-655-2877

    Website: *www.longevityformulas.com*

    E-mail: *info@longevityformulas.com*

Metagenics, Inc.: Committed to providing high-quality, innovative nutritional supplements at the best possible value for almost twenty years.

    100 Avenida La Pata; San Clemente, CA 92673

    Tel: 800-692-9400 or 949-366-0818

    Website: *www.metagenics.com*

NutriGuard Research: Carries arginine pyroglutamate, phosphatidylcholine, Staminex, glucosamine, and many multinutrient formulas.

> 1051 Hermes Avenue; Encinitas, CA 92024
> Tel: 800-433-2402
> From outside the U.S. and Canada, call 760-942-3223
> Website: *www.nutriguard.com*

Olympia Nutrition: A source for brain products like DMAE, acetylcarnitine, phosphatidylserine, MegaMind, NADH, DHEA, and hard-to-find products.

> 3579 Highway 50 East #220; Carson City, NV 89701
> Tel: 888-366-9909 or 775-887-7516
> Fax: 775-884-6042
> E-mail: *olympianet@aol.com*

PhytoPharmica: Manufactures more than 200 natural medicines, nutritional supplements, vitamins, and herbal extracts. Their product line is distributed exclusively through pharmacies and health care professionals nationwide.

> 825 Challenger Drive; Green Bay, WI 54311
> Tel: 800-553-2370
> Website: *www.phytopharmica.com*

Professional Complementary Health Formulas, PCHF: Provides products directly to health care practitioners—a wide variety of custom-made homeopathics for: desensitization, symptomatic and functional disturbances, the mind-body connection, drainage and energetic pharmacology, pathogenic disturbances, substances affecting the body of unnatural or man-made origin, a veterinary line for those conditions affecting animals, and cell salts. Their nutritionals include encapsulated New Zealand glandular combinations and single "pure" glands, amino acid complexes, herbal combinations, and Botanical Pure extracts.

> P.O. Box 80085; Portland, OR 97280
> Tel: 800-952-2219
> Website: *www.professionalformulas.com*
> E-mail: *pchf@professionalformulas.com*

River of Life Natural Foods: Stocks numerous smart nutrients including hard-to-find items and an extensive line of Source Naturals products.

> 5743 Lower York Road; Lahaska, PA 18931
> Tel: 800-651-3820 or 215-794-1445

Smartbomb.com: Sells TMG, NADH, 5-HTP, DMAE, DHEA, and a lot of other smart nutrient name-brand products from many companies.

320 South Street, Suite 11-H; Morristown, NJ 07960
Tel: 800-425-3115
Website: *www.smartbomb.com*
E-mail: *questions@smartbomb.com*

Smart Nutrition: Offers a broad range of cutting-edge nutritional supplements.

1765 Garnet Avenue #66; San Diego, CA 92109
Tel: 800-479-2107 or 619-270-9015
Fax: 800-349-8034
Website: *www.smart-drugs.com*
E-mail: *ias@smart-drugs.com*

Tierra Marketing International, TMI: A worldwide source for original, procaine-based Gerovital (GH3), 5-hydroxytryptophan, NADH, DHEA, and pregnenolone.

223 N. Guadalupe, Suite 285; Santa Fe, NM 87501
Tel: 800-736-6253
Fax: 505-982-0698
Website: *www.realgh3.com*
E-mail: *vitaman@rt66.com*

Transitions for Health, Inc.: Offers premium products, services, and information that can improve the health and lives of women. TFH is developing products designed for women, and they are dedicated to being an authoritative resource for women about wellness and vitality.

621 SW Alder Street, Suite 900; Portland, OR 97205
Tel: 800-648-8211 or 503-226-1010
Fax: 800-944-0168 or 503-226-6455
Website: *www.transitionsforhealth.com*

TriMedica, Inc.: A source for pregnenolone and DHEA.

1895 South Los Feliz Drive; Tempe, AZ 85281
Tel: 800-800-8849 (USA) or 480-988-1041 (elsewhere)
Fax: 480-998-1530
Website: *www.trimedica.com*
E-mail: *sales@trimedica.com*

Tyler, Inc.: Carries nutritionals and thyroid and adrenal supplements.
  2204 NW Birdsdale; Gresham, OR 97030
  Tel: 800-869-9705 or 503-661-5401
  Website: *www.tyler-inc.com*

Vitamin Express: Operates a chain of full-spectrum health food stores in the San Francisco Bay area with an extensive number of items; they mail worldwide.
  1428 Irving Street; San Francisco, CA 94122-2016
  Tel: 415-564-8160
  Fax (in SF store): 415-564-3156
  Website: *www.vitaminexpress.com*
  Branch locations: 1400 Shattuck Avenue, Berkeley, CA 94709 (Tel: 510-841-1798) and 45 Camino Alto, Mill Valley, CA 94901 (Tel: 415-389-9671)

Vitamin Research Products: VRP carries a complete line of dietary supplements. They sell powdered ingredients for do-it-yourselfers, take custom orders, and mail worldwide.
  3579 Highway 50 East; Carson City, NV 89701
  Tel: 800-877-2447 or 775-884-1300
  Fax: 800-877-3293 or 775-884-1331
  Website: *www.vrp.com*
  E-mail: *mail@vrp.com* or *customer.service@vrp.com*

VNF Nutrition: Specializes in natural products and is committed to representing manufacturers of only high-quality natural products, including vitamins, supplements, herbal products, and natural body-care items.
  246 Rt. 25A; Setauket, NY 11733
  Tel: 800-681-7099 or 631-689-6433
  Int. Tel: 011-631-689-0690
  Fax: 631-689-7638
  Website: *www.vnfnutrition.com*
  E-mail: *vnf@vnfnutrition.com*

Western Research Laboratories: Another source for natural thyroid Rx.
  21602 North 21st Avenue; Phoenix, AZ 85027
  Tel: 877-797-7997
  Fax: 623-879-8683
  Website: *www.westernresearchlaboratories.com*

International Resources

For an extensive list of overseas pharmacies, smart drugs, and anti-aging products and information, go to: *http://qualitycounts.com/stores/overseas.html*

Era-Bond Laboratories: Carries GHB and other popular smart and prosexual drugs such as bromocriptine, deprenyl, DHEA, L-Dopa, hydergine, melatonin, metformin, piracetam, tryptophan, vincamine.
    72 New Bond Street; London W1Y 9DD; United Kingdom
    Fax: 011-44-207-499-3417

Masters Marketing Company, Ltd.: Provides European pharmaceuticals and nutritional supplements. They have a long-standing reputation for excellent service.
    Masters House, 5 Sandridge Close; Harrow HA1 1TW; United Kingdom
    Tel: 011-44-208-424-9400
    Fax: 011-44-208-427-1994
    Website: *www.mastersmedical.com*
    E-mail: *info@mastersmedical.com*
    (in USA) Masters Medical, Inc.; 10218 NW 50th Street; Sunrise, FL 33351

Quality Health, Inc.: Offers the most popular smart drugs as well as L-tryptophan and a range of nutritional supplements.
    401 Langham House; 29-30 Margaret Street; London W1W 8SA;
        United Kingdom
    Tel: 011-44-207-580-2043
    Fax: 011-44-207-580-2043
    Information voice mail for U.S. and Canadian customers: 888-594-4555
    Website: *www.qhi.co.uk*
    E-mail: *sales@qhi.co.uk*

Victoria Apotheke Zurich: A mail-order source well known for locating hard-to-find pharmaceuticals for those contending with life-threatening diseases. They also carry a wide range of smart drugs and life-extension items. On-line catalog available.
    Bahnhofstrasse 71; Postfach, CH-8021 Zurich; Switzerland
    Tel: 011-411-211-2432
    Fax: 011-411-221-2322
    Website: *www.pharmaworld.com*
    E-mail: *info@pharmaworld.com*
    Pharmacist: Dr. C. Eglof, Ph.D.

GLOSSARY OF REMEDIES

As "provings" for new homeopathic remedies continue, extensive resources expand. The following abbreviated glossary includes specific pictures common to remedies relevant to conditions presented throughout the book; others are listed with certain conditions, especially in Chapter 6. As each remedy, herb, or formula has many properties, for more details, please refer to books listed in the Bibliography.

HOMEOPATHIC REMEDIES

Individual Remedies (If known, consider your constitutional remedy as your first line of defense.)

Aconite stops uterine hemorrhage accompanied by an enormous fear of impending death.

Antimonium Crudum is for the woman who tends to be soft and quiet, sensitive and emotional, sweet and sad, with a pleasant round face. She loves food and loves to eat, often craving sour foods like pickles. Those same foods may cause digestive disturbances like diarrhea, or alternating diarrhea and constipation.

Apis is for the woman on the go who can be very sensible and business-minded. Being task-oriented, she tends toward being a workaholic. When it comes to family affairs, she controls and reveals jealousy. Her key emotional issue inclines to be irritability. The Apis woman develops right ovarian cysts with her endometriosis, along with severe dysmenorrhea. If she does conceive, she is likely to spontaneously miscarry in the first trimester. She may also experience cystitis-like symptoms cyclically. Her sex drive may increase, but she normally maintains a healthy and balanced sex life. Apis relieves the intensity associated with the almost violent downward-pressure pain and dark mucousy blood. Some women actually feel as if they're in labor when their menses begins.

Argentum Metallicum is for the woman who usually seems fairly extroverted, even impulsive, and expresses herself with ease. Her ovarian pain arrives suddenly.

Aurum is for the woman who is very intense and idealistic; she can drop into the depths of despair when devastated by grief. Aurum helps when her sex drive is altered by grief or suicidal ideation.

Belladonna is for the woman who is usually balanced and healthy yet experiences sudden acute conditions. Along with her fever, she may develop hallucinations or delirium. Belladonna helps stop uterine hemorrhage, especially when the bleeding is bright red and feels hot, and pelvic pain that makes her feel as if her entire pelvis is trying to push itself out through a bearing-down sensation. It can help with hormonal headaches and migraines. This woman experiences her mastitis with deep redness to the affected area. Her breast is hot to the touch—almost the feeling of being scalded—and marked with much inflammation, and she has significant tenderness with an intense throbbing or pulsing sensation. When she develops an ovarian cyst, it is with sudden onset, and her pain is worse before or during her period; the intensity of her ovarian pain is exacerbated by any movement. The skin of the pelvic region covering the affected ovary may feel hot to the touch, marked with the sensation of much inflammation. She has significant tenderness with an intense throbbing or pulsing sensation. Bright red bleeding accompanies the rupture of a cyst.

Bryonia is for the woman who is quite focused on core survival issues; she is business-oriented with the need to work hard to cover the cost of living. She will be quite irritable and prefer solitude when she develops mastitis. Her fever comes on slowly, though it can rise high as with the Belladonna picture. As her condition worsens over several days, her breast becomes hard and hot. The slightest movement intensifies her pain and even though she may feel agitated, she will try to lie very still on the affected side, more often on the right.

Calcarea Carbonica is also a commonly used constitutional remedy. Often exhausted from working hard, the responsible Calc Carb woman is overworked, overloaded, overinundated, exhausted, anxious about her health, and tends to gain weight with great ease. She craves sweets, pastries, ice cream, milk, cheeses, and salty foods. Digestive disturbances may plague her along with constipation. Calcarea Carbonica can help with hypothyroidism in one who tends to be chilly and gets cold easily, while also easily gaining weight. Her symptoms worsen when she feels cold. It also helps with metrorrhagia in menopause. Her breasts swell, sometimes feeling hot, and become quite painful before her menses. If her milk supply was abundant while nursing, it may at times have been disagreeable to her baby, and continues to be excessive after weaning (galactorrhea). Also common to the woman who needs Calc Carb are swollen and painful breasts, predominantly before her menses.

Carbo Animalis is for the woman who experiences everything worse during her menses; she feels weak and lacking in her vital sense of well-being. She develops fibrocystic breasts, breast abscesses, breast tumors, or breast cysts. Her breast conditions tend to emerge on her left side. The need for Carbo Animalis often accompanies the appearance of malignancy or actual malignancy. If this woman develops breast cancer, according to Roger Morrison, M.D., "the cancer grows slowly with progressing masses which burn or sting and may have offensive discharges and enlarged axillary nodes."

Carbo Vegetabilis is for the woman who often presents with weak digestion, distension, and bloating. She also tends to long for sweets and salty foods or seems unresponsive to food altogether. Conversely, she may approach food with voracity.

Caulophyllum, primarily used in pregnancy, supports functional labor, helps arrest excessive bleeding postpartum and in metrorrhagia. It can help prevent early miscarriage, or support a healthier passing of the fetus if miscarriage is unavoidable. It has also been used in infertility.

Causticum is for aversion to coition, often with vaginal/bladder burning, and is a commonly used remedy with bladder infections and symptoms associated with burning sensations.

Chamomilla can relieve your mood when you feel impatient and your fuse remains short, independent of excess sugar or caffeine, and it alleviates cramps.

China Officinalis is for the introverted type who experiences dark blood with her heavy flow, along with digestive disturbances and gallbladder symptoms.

Conium has been one of the main remedies to resist malignant and premalignant conditions, and has been used to help treat breast cancer, often with axillary lymph node involvement, according to William Boericke, M.D., Roger Morrison, M.D., and other renowned homeopathic physicians. It is also used to treat cyclic cystic breast conditions. Conium assists with marked sexual dysfunction.

Crocus Sativus is for the woman who often experiences hysteria and suffers uterine hemorrhage with dark, stringy clots.

Ferrum is for the woman who flushes easily with rosy cheeks from a circulatory dysfunction and floods with her excessive bleeding. She desires sweets, bread, and butter. Insatiable or uninterested in food, she may experience abdominal pains with repositioning her body. Ferrum is utilized to strengthen defenses.

Graphites is for the woman who is described as an earthy, peasant type in appearance. She tends toward constipation and prefers bland, simple foods—chicken, beer, and sometimes sweets. Graphites assists when there is an aversion to sex.

Helonias focuses on female hormonal issues and uterine dysfunctions. The woman who will benefit from Helonias has an awareness of her womb all the time, feeling changes in its position as she moves.

Hepar Sulphur is for the woman who is exquisitely sensitive to pain, especially as it increases her sense of vulnerability; this woman develops mastitis and/or breast abscesses.

Ignatia helps move the grief out of our cells, out of our bodies. Every woman I have ever met with a history of endometriosis, miscarriage, and many other conditions specific to the female body and psyche has experienced grief.

Ipecacuanha is primarily a remedy for nausea and vomiting; it arrests sudden onset, bright red gushing blood, without clots, along with nausea, vomiting, and fainting. The heavy bleeding is worse upon motion and postpartum. The woman who will benefit from Ipecacuanha experiences severe dysmenorrhea with nausea. It can be used in threatened miscarriages, especially with nausea and vomiting.

Kali Bichromicum is for the woman who conforms, clinging to her beliefs as well as her routines. She will yearn for sweets and lean toward diarrhea or colitis. Pain may radiate from her left-sided cyst, though not always. This woman feels like an unlucky victim abandoned by God. She tends to be highly sexual with uterine fibroids more on the right side.

Kali Carbonicum is for the woman who is conservative, proper, dogmatic, and avoids change. She loves sweets and becomes constipated just prior to or with her menses. Along with uterine fibroids, she may experience bleeding between menses or skip them altogether.

Kali Ferrocyanatum is for the woman who may experience profuse, painless hemorrhaging, taking her into radical anemia. She likely has uterine fibroids.

Kali Iodatum assists with both hypothyroidism and hyperthyroidism, with or without the presence of a goiter.

Lac Caninum is for the woman with a significant sensitivity to sound, light, and touch. She shares some of the extroverted qualities of Phosphorus, and her imagination tends toward hysteria and many fears. Before her menses, she likely develops painful, swollen breasts, which worsen if she is bumped or jolted.

Lachesis is for the woman who is highly passionate and intense in all aspects of her life. She seems to sustain an extreme inner irritability that is interwoven with her intensity and often her loquaciousness. She loves with the same intensity and passion she brings to everything else, maintaining high sexual energy. When she is unable to effectively express her ardor, these aspects of her personality become suppressed and she seems introverted. Her endometriosis more often affects her left ovary along with severe dysmenorrhea, during which clothing, especially anything restrictive from the waist down, is unbearable. She is likely to seek escape with alcohol or drugs as the intensity of her grief and debilitating pain overwhelms her. Her PMS symptoms are classically extreme with irritability, jealousy bordering on paranoia, depression intermittent with angry outbursts, increased anxiety, headaches, and at times she contemplates suicide. If she is backed into a corner, she can strike with the same piercing and venomous bite as a snake. Unable to lie on her left side, she will sleep on her right. Her left ovary may pulsate with pain from the cyst.

Lycopodium is for the woman who tends toward a lack of self-confidence and self-esteem. Often she's more introverted and a shy loner. She can also exhibit the opposite to compensate for her feeling of inadequacy. Even though she develops right-sided ovarian cysts, she continues to sleep only on that side. She may have fine features and hold her extra pounds in her buttocks and around her thighs, giving meaning to the term *love handles*. She has frequent digestive disturbances, though she enjoys sweets and has an insatiable appetite.

Natrum Muriaticum is for the woman who grieves and becomes emotionally shut down, developing an aversion to sex. She usually experiences painful intercourse as a result of vaginal dryness.

Nux Vomica is for the classic workaholic with the type A personality, to the max. She is impatient and literally hates to wait for anything, and waiting can drive her into an agitated state. She is easily offended and angered by contradiction. Perhaps her greatest fear is failure, so she focuses intensely on her work with a fierce competitive ambitiousness—she must win. Her sense of self depends on it. She loves coffee, she loves alcohol, she loves spicy foods, perhaps tobacco as well, and anything else that stimulates her senses. She can be promiscuous to satisfy her high sex drive, but not always. Her endometriosis may involve her lower bowel, causing her posterior pressure or an urge to pass stool with the onset of her dysmenorrhea. Her pain—uterine, lower back, sometimes including bladder involvement—tends to be spastic and congested. Nux Vomica is another good remedy for irritable PMS.

Onosmodium is for the woman who has a preoccupation with sex and loss of libido, headaches or migraines with eyestrain.

Palladium, another woman's remedy, is primarily used to treat right-sided ovarian cysts with pain that worsens with sudden movement or excitement. Relief comes from lying on her left side.

Phosphorus is for the woman who bubbles with her own excitement and enthusiasm, with virtually no boundaries around others and who often seems ungrounded, lacking an anchor or centeredness. This is a good remedy for fibrocystic breasts.

Phytolacca is a glandular-focused remedy, assisting with fibrocystic breasts, characterized by painful breasts before and during menses, and painful benign breast lumps. It has also been known to palliate breast cancer, though not cure it.

Platinum is for the woman who exudes arrogance and seems to feel superior to others, as though she is of royal blood. If she is not egotistical, she diverts her passionate nature toward her sexuality. Along with intense dysmenorrhea, frequently accompanied by a bearing-down sensation, she develops left-sided ovarian cysts.

Plumbum helps prevent miscarriage and works on neurological and circulatory systems.

Pulsatilla is for the woman who presents as a soft, gentle, even meek individual who needs strong people around to dominate or influence her; she is more commonly blond and fair-skinned, plump with flushed cheeks and red lips, but not always. She is warm and feels worse from heat, and she loves to eat butter, cheeses, creamy foods, and sweets. Rich and fatty foods cause her indigestion. Shy, she seems dependent, emotional—crying easily, sensitive, sympathetic, and feels better with consolation, especially by someone she respects as an authority. Though highly sexed, she may develop an absolute aversion to sex, especially if she has surrendered her sexual drive to a fervent religious belief system that does not support sexuality, especially in women. Her sex drive is fueled by her strong desire for a deep emotional connection with another. Her mood swings change from the extreme of weeping one moment to intense irritability the next, particularly if she feels forsaken, deprived, or needs attention. Pulsatilla treats galactorrhea, mastitis, and fibrocystic breasts. The intense dysmenorrhea begins at a young age, often from the beginning of her cycles at menarche. Her menses may be shorter than the unusual picture of endometriosis, but they tend to be heavy and just as exquisitely painful, with the pain more pronounced in her lower left abdominal side.

Sabina, a primary remedy for uterine problems, helps to stop hemorrhages accompanied by intense pain, active gushing, and often accompanied by clots and a bright red flow. Ideal for the woman who may experience bleeding between her menses, which can be made worse from uterine fibroids. This woman experiences uterine pain from dysmenorrhea as well as other uterine disorders. Her pain may begin in her lower back, sacrum, and expand to her pubis.

Sepia may be confused with Pulsatilla because the woman for whom this is appropriate cries easily, often weeping for no known reason, only she (Sepia) tends to be brunette. She appears to have a harder edge, more indifferent than sympathetic. She often feels disconnected and isolated from others, so much so that her previous preoccupation with guilty feelings turns into a cutting detachment at another's weakness, intuited and expressed with acute and unkind accuracy. Her symptoms are more severely perceived on her left side, accompanied by an intense bearing-down sensation as though her uterus will prolapse and fall out, particularly during her painful menstrual flow. Her PMS is marked with irritability to the point of yelling at her loved ones, significant depression, and weeping despairingly. She experiences aggravation from her hormonal imbalance and from coition, and sex becomes so painful (dyspareunia) that she may develop an actual aversion not only to sex but also to being touched. Infertility is common, but if she does conceive after she has developed endometriosis, she is more likely to miscarry in the first trimester. Other tendencies for the Sepia woman, which suggest a need for immune support, include herpes, genital warts, psoriasis, and chronic fatigue syndrome (CFS). Her circulation may show cold hands and feet, or Raynaud's disease.

Silica is for the woman who is described as refined, delicate, responsive, and acquiescent. Although generally balanced, she lacks self-esteem. As a nursing mother, she develops mastitis. She can have a tendency toward fibrocystic breasts. Silica also treats breast abscesses and nodules.

Tarentula Hispanica is for the woman who tends to be highly sexual, her nervous system overstimulated, even hyperactive. She often experiences bleeding between her normal cycles and may experience a burning sensation in her uterus.

Thuja is for the woman who lacks self-esteem and often feels unattractive, lonely, and sad from her inability to fit in. She can develop uterine tumors, with a tendency toward fibroids, as well as ovarian cysts, on her left side.

Ustilago is said by several homeopaths to treat left-sided swollen ovaries with a burning type of pain. This pain may radiate down into the woman's legs.

Combination Formulas

Aletris-Heel relieves symptoms of exhaustion and weakness following overexertion.

Apo-Strum, a combination, low-potency formula in an alcohol base produced by PEKANA, a German pharmaceutical company, is indicated for treatment of thyroid dysfunctions, including hardening or enlargement of the thyroid gland.

BHI Calming soothes restlessness, irritability, melancholy, and helps with insomnia.

BHI Exhaustion is recommended for fatigue and exhaustion following exertion, overwork, stress, insomnia, and for during or following illness.

BHI Feminine is for difficult and irregular menses, pelvic pain, vaginal dryness after menses, and hot flashes.

BHI Liver helps with liver congestion and related symptoms.

Cardinorma taken as 20 drops three times a day, treats cardiac insufficiency, tachycardia, cardiac spasms, circulatory conditions, and increases oxygen utilization.

China-Homaccord helps with the relief of fatigue and exhaustion caused by stress, overwork, and chronic illness.

Co-Hypert—15 to 20 drops three times a day—helps to reduce and regulate high blood pressure.

Coro-Calm is a cardiac sedative taken 15 to 20 drops three times a day to treat tachycardia, disrupted circulatory functions, pulse abnormalities; it improves oxygenation and calms the nervous response to these conditions.

Galium-Heel assists in increasing the activation of the body's defense mechanisms.

Hormeel helps regulate irregular menstrual cycles and reduces bloating and nervous irritability.

Klifem drops work to regulate menstrual irregularities, the tendency to obesity in menopause, hot flashes, night sweats, and breast tenderness.

Klimaktheel helps relieve hot flashes, excessive swelling and edema, headaches, fatigue, and irritability.

Nervoheel relieves symptoms of stress, restlessness, insomnia, and nervous tension.

Selenium-Homaccord assists with stress-related mental fatigue and the inability to concentrate.

Somcupin, taken 20 drops three times a day and at bedtime, deals directly with both the physical and psychic factors leading to insomnia and sleep disturbances.

Valerianaheel, taken 10 drops three times a day and at bedtime, relieves nervous anxiety, restlessness, nervous exhaustion, and insomnia.

Ypsiloheel is indicated for stress and nervous irritability.

HERBAL REMEDIES

Chinese Herbals (Descriptions are based on Golden Flower Chinese Herbs Formula Guide, except for those indicated*.)

Beauty Pearl* assists with PMS symptoms through the focus of balancing hormones.

Bupleurum and Tang Kuei Formula regulates and harmonizes the energy of the liver and spleen, specifically to help with tenderness, distension, lumps, and fibrocystic tendencies in the breasts, bloating, depression, emotional instability, irritability, moodiness, fatigue, headaches, dizziness, irregular cycles, and menstrual cramps. It also helps with heavy and irregular bleeding and assists with other menopausal symptoms. This formula should not be used if you have abdominal distension or signs of excess heat defined by excessive vital function demonstrating feverishness, flushed face, thirst with the desire for cold drinks, constipation, a rapid pulse, and reddening of the tongue with a yellowish coating.

Cinnamon plus Dragon Bone and Oyster Formula regulates and helps balance yin and yang, and is used for physical symptoms from chronic constraint, overwork, and other psychological issues.

Dong Quai*, taken in a tincture of 15 to 20 drops four times a day for up to seven days, can induce a late menses and temporarily relieve the edginess of PMS. Prolonged usage of dong quai alone can potentiate heavy bleeding. It is commonly found in many women's formulas.

Free and Easy Wanderer Plus assists with increased anxiety, angry outbursts, depression, irritability, restlessness, emotional instability, as well as breast pain, swelling, and lumps; menstrual nausea and vomiting; and irregular and painful periods. Do not take this if you think you might be pregnant.

Gingerroot Tea* soothes, nourishes, and relieves cramping and helps with irregular bleeding.

Ginseng and Astragalus Formula supports your central qi as it tonifies stomach and spleen qi. While it replenishes the qi, it raises depressed yang energy.

Ginseng Nourishing Formula is a nutritive combination of herbs especially good if you lack vitality. It nourishes the heart, calms the spirit, and sharpens the memory.

Heavenly Emperor's Formula is considered an herbal alternative to tranquilizers and sleeping pills. It assists with forgetfulness and the inability to focus with mental clarity.

Salvia Ten Formula assists with accompanying depression as it supports general vitality and soothes the nerves.

Sea of Qi Formula slows prolonged menstruation and warms and tonifies.

Tang Kuei and Peony Formula focuses on balancing physical PMS symptoms.

Western Herbs

Black Cohosh calms hysteria and relieves cramps.

Black Currant, taken 15 to 20 drops three times a day, helps prevent urinary infections while it nourishes the adrenal glands.

Chasteberry, demonstrating phytoestrogenic qualities, lessens breast pain, fluid retention, headaches, and fatigue. It appears to help increase progesterone.

Cinnamon, taken 20 drops twice a day, helps regulate cycles; taken 10 drops every fifteen to twenty minutes will slow flooding.

Corn Silk Tea soothes the bladder. Drink copious amounts freely throughout the day. Shuck ears of corn and separate the silken threads. Steep the threads in boiled water. Corn silk is also available in herbal capsules if corn is out of season.

Cramp Bark relaxes nerves and relieves cramps and spasms.

Damiana, taken 375 mg one to three times a day, acts as a diuretic; it also acts directly on the reproductive system and as an aphrodisiac.

Dandelion Root helps with cramps and constipation; 10 to 25 drops before meals relieves digestive distress.

Devil's Club, taken 5 to 20 drops three times a day, evens blood sugar, alleviates constipation, and is beneficial with hot flashes.

Evening Primrose Oil, a natural source of the fatty acid gamma-linolenic acid, helps relieve menstrual cramps, breast swelling, lumps, and pain.

Fenugreek Seeds, one tablespoon per cup of water boiled for ten minutes, makes a lovely tea that helps digestion, stabilizes blood sugar, and sweetens the fragrance of your sweat.

Feverfew is an anti-inflammatory herb that also stimulates the uterus and helps with headaches.

Ginseng, taken 5 to 20 drops three times a day, relieves indigestion, reduces fatigue, decreases hot flashes, and can soothe anxiety and depression.

Lady's Mantle, taken 10 drops three times a day for one to two weeks before menses, helps control hemorrhaging and prevent flooding. It may cause contractions of the uterus.

Licorice Root contains phytoestrogenic properties and is an antiviral and alleviates cramps. Licorice root contains glycyrrhizin acid, a readily available inhibitor of the enzyme that deactivates cortisol and helps sustain cortisol levels. High doses of licorice can have negative side effects such as high blood pressure and water retention.

Nettle Leaf Tea: drink a cup a day to help regulate flow and support adrenals.

Oregon Grape Root, 150 mg, helps to purify the blood, and in combination with 30 mg of cascara sagrada bark assists in digestion and absorption, as well as constipation, although, I think cascara sagrada can be a rather harsh herb.

Panax Ginseng and Siberian Ginseng increase our resistance to stress factors and enhance adrenal function.

Sarsaparilla, taken 500 mg a day a week or two before your period, has diuretic qualities if you suffer from fluid retention.

Shepherd's Purse, taken 20 drops four times a day, decreases heavy bleeding; taken 15 to 20 drops held under the tongue four to six times a day relieves flooding.

Uva Ursi, taken 10 to 20 drops three to six times a day for one to two days, then three times a day for up to ten days, helps heal infections.

Vitex, taken 20 drops three times a day, assists with menstrual irregularities.

Wild Yam Root, uncompounded, 200 mg a day, can stimulate your body to increase its progesterone production, and can also be taken 20 drops three to four times a day for midcycle spotting. But it is not as effective as compounded phytogenic progesterone.

Witch Hazel, taken 20 drops four times a day, is said to tonify the uterus and promote normal menses.

Yarrow Tea helps tonify the bladder as well as fight infection. Drink once or twice a day.

VITAMINS AND MINERALS

Antioxidants are natural chemical compounds that slow or prevent oxygen from reacting with other compounds, some of which demonstrate cancer-protecting potential because they neutralize free radicals. Examples include vitamins C and E, beta-carotene, the minerals selenium and germanium, superoxide dismutase (SOD), coenzyme Q10, catalase, and some amino acids.

Beta-carotene, the most abundant of the carotenoids, provides strong pro–vitamin A activity, is a stronger antioxidant than vitamin A, and is a cancer preventative. Found in leafy green and yellow vegetables, beta-carotene is an excellent source for your body to convert into vitamin A when you need it.

Boron assists in the absorption and utilization of calcium; when mixed with the B vitamins, the effect of the calcium and the Bs soothes the nervous system.

Calcium, the most abundant mineral in the body, is necessary for bone and tooth development, prevents muscle cramps, and helps to promote blood clotting. Calcium requires hydrochloric acid, magnesium, and vitamins D, E, and C for adequate absorption.

Choline, a lipotropic substance found in vitamin B complex, is essential for the metabolism of fats in the body; as a precursor to acetylcholine, it is a major neurotransmitter in the brain. Deficiency leads to cirrhosis of the liver.

Copper, an essential mineral found in all body tissues, when deficient causes abnormalities such as anemia, skeletal defects, degeneration of the nervous system, reproductive failure, pronounced cardiovascular lesions, elevated blood cholesterol, impaired immunity, and defects in the pigmentation and structure of hair. Copper is associated with iron incorporation into hemoglobin, and with vitamin C in the formation of collagen and the correct functioning of the central nervous system. Copper contains many enzymes.

Docosahexaenoic acid (DHA) is a metabolite of the omega-3 fatty acid alpha-linolenic acid.

Fatty acids are chemical chains of carbon, hydrogen, and oxygen atoms, part of a lipid (fat) and the significant aspect of triglycerides. Fatty acids are classified as either saturated, polyunsaturated, or monounsaturated.

Folic acid, a part of vitamin B complex, functions along with vitamins B-12 and C in the utilization of proteins, and is essential in the formation of DNA and heme, the iron-containing protein in hemoglobin necessary for the formation of red blood cells. Essential during pregnancy, folic acid prevents neural tubular defects in the developing fetus.

Glutathione peroxidase, a group of antioxidant enzymes that contain selenium, is important in the reduction of gastrointestinal tract irritation.

Iodine is an essential mineral vital to the thyroid hormones, thyroxin and triiodothyronine. Iodine deficiencies can result in development of a goiter, reduced vitality, and hypothyroidism and its associated symptoms.

Iron is required by hemoglobin, without which red blood cells could not live. Our bodies must absorb iron (ferrous compounds) as a salt—such as ferrous gluconate, carbonate, sulfate, or fumerate along with vitamin C to enable this absorption.

Magnesium is an essential mineral whose chief function is to activate certain enzymes, especially those related to carbohydrate metabolism. It maintains the electrical potential across nerve and muscle membranes, and is essential for proper heartbeat and nerve transmission. Magnesium controls many cellular functions; is involved in protein formation and DNA production and function; and helps the storage and release of energy in adenosine triphosphate (ATP). Magnesium is closely related to calcium and phosphorus in body function.

Melatonin, the only hormone secreted into the bloodstream by the pineal gland, appears to inhibit numerous endocrine functions. Melatonin supplements treat some insomnia and sleep disturbances and jet lag. Dosages higher than 1 mg may cause drowsiness or headaches and may alter normal circadian rhythms. It is contraindicated in those who are on antidepressant and insulin medication, and may have a negative influence on estrogen production.

Methionine, an essential amino acid and antioxidant nutrient, is important for proper growth in infants and nitrogen balance in adults; it promotes the physiological utilization of fat, healthy nails and skin, and the synthesis of lecithin, bile, and endorphins.

Pantothenic acid is a B complex vitamin necessary for the normal functioning of the adrenal gland, which directly affects growth; it is also essential for the formation of fatty acids, and as a coenzyme it participates in the utilization of riboflavin and in the release of energy from carbohydrates, fats, and proteins.

Para-aminobenzoic acid (PABA) is considered part of the vitamin B complex; as a coenzyme, PABA functions in the breakdown and utilization of proteins and in the formation of red blood cells.

Potassium is a mineral that serves as an electrolyte and is involved in the balance of fluid within the body.

Selenium, an essential element primarily in antioxidant enzymes, assists in thyroid hormone production, lowers the risk of several types of cancers, and, in combination with vitamin E, augments the production of antibodies, the maintenance of a healthy heart, the function of the pancreas, and the elasticity of tissues, and enhances cellular defense against oxidation damage.

Tryptophan, an essential amino acid, is a natural relaxant and sleep aid because it is a precursor in serotonin synthesis. In combination with tyrosine, it has been helpful in treating addictions.

Vitamin A maintains the integrity of cilia, tiny threadlike hairs in the fallopian tubes and elsewhere. Vitamin A is as responsible for fertility as is vitamin E. It also affects the dryness and texture of our skin, including our labia.

Vitamin Bs calm the nervous system; affect some mental symptoms of depression and confusion; are necessary to assist in the metabolization of fats, proteins, carbohydrates, and amino acids; have an anti–gray hair factor and antianemic qualities.

Vitamin B-3, niacin, found in vitamin B complex, helps facilitate the breakdown of carbohydrates, fats, and proteins. Found in every cell of the body, niacin is necessary for energy production, DNA formation, and the health of the skin, nerves, tongue, and digestive system.

Vitamin B-6, pyridoxine, influences many body functions, including the regulation of blood glucose levels and the manufacture of hemoglobin, and aids the utilization of protein, carbohydrates, and fats. It also aids in the function of the nervous system.

Vitamin B-15, pangamic acid, helps regulate the hypothalamus, pituitary, and adrenal axis. It also eliminates jet lag.

Vitamin C, also known as **ascorbic acid,** is a water-soluble antioxidant essential for the maintenance of bones, teeth, collagen, and blood vessels (capillaries); it inhibits the formation of nitrosamines (a suspected carcinogen), enhances iron absorption and red blood cell formation, and helps in the utilization of carbohydrates and the synthesis of fats and proteins.

Vitamin D, a fat-soluble vitamin, is necessary for normal assimilation of calcium and phosphorus to maintain healthy bone formation, mineralization, and tooth development. Vitamin D is a prohormone with several active metabolites that act as hormones, and it occurs mainly in two forms: ergocalciferol (activated ergosterol, vitamin D_2), found in irradiated yeast; and cholecalciferol (activated 7-dehydrocholesterol, vitamin D_3), formed in human skin by exposure to sunlight (ultraviolet radiation) and found chiefly in fish liver oils and egg yolks. Both can also be found in carrots. One microgram of vitamin D equals 40 IU.

Vitamin E, an antioxidant, protects tissue, helps with muscle repair, and effects electron transfer—when one electron leaves an element to join another element. As vitamin E is necessary to maintain each muscular system, including the uterus, it also stimulates the production of our female hormones; so, via both of these mechanisms, vitamin E helps decrease cramps and even out hormone levels. Another function of vitamin E is to stimulate the thyroid.

Zinc is an essential trace mineral with enzymatic functions for more than seventy metalloenzymes, protein synthesis, and carbohydrate metabolism. Zinc supports the health of immune function, assists vitamin A utilization, and is involved in the formation of bone and teeth.

AROMATHERAPY

In addition to the following, which contain some phytohormonal properties, there are many other essential oils used in aromatherapy that you can explore in a specialty shop or check into at websites; go to, for example, *www.frontier coop.com/Auracacia/* or *www.youngliving.com*

Bergamot (*Citrus bergamia*) has an aroma that is fresh, lively, fruity, and sweet—a lovely deodorizer—and produces the aromatherapy benefits of up-lifting, inspiring, and helping to build self-confidence.

Cedarwood (*Cedrus atlantica*) gives off a woody, oily scent that is sometimes described as slightly animal-like, with the aromatherapy values of stabiliz-ing, centering, and strengthening the mind and mood.

Cinnamon bark (*Cinnamomum zeylanicum*) permeates with a warm, spicy effect and gives the aromatherapy benefits of comforting and warming.

Clary sage (*Salvia sclarea*) generates a spicy, bittersweet aroma with the aroma-therapy benefits of centering, euphoria, and enhancing visualization.

Fennel, sweet (*Foeniculum vulgare var. dulce*) emits a sweet, earthy, aniselike aroma, and offers the aromatherapy qualities of nurturing, supporting, and restoring.

Geranium (*Pelargonium graveolens*) releases a powerful, roselike fragrance with fruity, mint undertones; the aromatherapy benefits are soothing, lifting moods, and balancing.

Ginger (*Zingiber officinale*) has a warm, spicy, woody odor, with the aroma-therapy effects of warming, strengthening, and anchoring.

Jasmine (*Jasminum grandiflorum*) emanates a full, rich, honeylike sweetness, sensual and romantic, with the aromatherapy benefits of calming and relax-ing.

Lavender (*Lavandula angustifolia*) exudes a sweet, balsamic, floral scent with the aromatherapy benefits of balancing, soothing, normalizing, calming, re-laxing, and healing.

Neroli (*Citrus aurantium*) has a very strong, refreshing, spicy, floral aroma with the aromatherapy benefits of calming and soothing, as well as sensual quali-ties.

Sandalwood (*Santalum album*) has a sweet-woody, warm, balsamic aroma with the aromatherapy benefits of relaxing, centering, and sensuality.

GLOSSARY OF TERMS

Abscess: A pocket of pus that forms as the body's defenses attempt to wall off infection-causing germs.

Adaptogenic: A substance or agent that facilitates adaptation; is usually nourishing and tonifying.

Addison's disease: Characterized by the chronic destruction of the adrenal cortex, leading to an increased loss of sodium and water in the urine, muscle weakness, and low blood pressure. The skin pigment melanin increases its production, causing a bronze color of the skin.

Allergy: Hypersensitivity caused by exposure to a particular antigen (allergen), resulting in an increased reactivity to that antigen on subsequent exposure, sometimes with harmful immunologic consequences.

Amino acid: An organic acid containing nitrogen chemical building blocks that aid in the production of protein in the body. Of the twenty-two known amino acids, eight are considered essential and must be obtained from dietary sources.

Anemia: A condition resulting from an unusually low number of red blood cells or too little hemoglobin in the red blood cells. Iron-deficiency anemia reduces the size and number of red blood cells, resulting in low hemoglobin levels. Clinical symptoms include shortness of breath, lethargy, and heart palpitations.

Anhydrous: Water deficient.

Antibody: A type of serum protein (globulin) synthesized by white blood cells of the lymphoid type in response to an antigenic (foreign substance) stimulus; normally fights infection.

Antigen: A protein or protein-sugar complex that, being foreign to the bloodstream or tissues, stimulates the formation of specific blood-serum antibodies and white-blood-cell activity.

Anxiety: Apprehension and possibly unexplained feelings/fears of danger or dread, accompanied by nervous restlessness and tension, increased heart rate, and shortness of breath.

Areola: The colored tissue that encircles the nipple.

Arrhythmia: A variation in the regular rhythm of the heartbeat; may cause serious conditions such as shock and congestive heart failure; can lead to death.

Aspiration: Removal of fluid from a cyst or cells from a lump, using a needle and syringe.

Atypical hyperplasia: Cells that are both abnormal (atypical) and increased in number. Benign microscopic breast changes known as atypical hyperplasia moderately increase a woman's risk of developing breast cancer.

Autoimmune disease: Conditions identified when the immune system rebels against the body's own cells, tissues, and organs, leading to chronic and potentially fatal results.

Average risk (for breast cancer): A measure of the chances of getting breast cancer without the presence of any specific factors known to be associated with the disease.

Ayurveda: Means the "science of life" and is a specific healing modality that originated in India more than five thousand years ago.

Benign: Not cancerous, it cannot invade neighboring tissues or spread to other parts of the body.

Benign breast changes: Noncancerous changes in the breast. Benign breast conditions can cause pain, lumpiness, nipple discharge, and other problems.

Bioavailable: Nutrients taken into the human body that do not require conversion to another form or source in order to be absorbed and utilized inside the body.

Bioflavonoids: Required for vitamin C absorption, they are found in fruits and vegetables.

Bioidentical: Nonhuman molecules that are indistinguishable in structure to those same molecules found biologically in the human body.

Biopsy: The removal of a sample of tissue or cells for examination under a microscope for purposes of diagnosis.

Blood deficiency: A Chinese medical term referring to presentations such as a pale or sallow complexion, pale lips, a pale tongue, and thready pulse, along with other symptoms including blurred vision, insomnia, dizziness, poor memory, and heart palpitations.

BRCA1 and BRCA2 genes: The principal genes that, when altered, indicate an inherited susceptibility to breast cancer. These gene alterations are present in 80 to 90 percent of hereditary cases of breast cancer.

Breast density: Glandular tissue in the breast common in younger women, making it difficult for mammography to detect breast cancer.

Breast implants: Silicone rubber sacs, filled with silicone gel or sterile saline, that are used for breast reconstruction after mastectomy or for cosmetic enhancement.

Calcifications: Small deposits of calcium in tissue, which can be seen on mammograms.

Cancer: A general name for more than one hundred diseases in which abnormal cells grow out of control. Cancer cells can invade and destroy healthy tissues, and they can spread to other parts of the body through the bloodstream and the lymphatic system.

Carcinoma: Cancer that begins in tissues lining or covering the surfaces (epithelial tissues) of organs, glands, or other body structures.

Carcinoma in situ: Cancer that is confined to the cells where it began and has not spread into surrounding tissues.

Chakra: Focalized energy points throughout the body. There are nine primary chakras and twenty-seven (to my knowledge) subchakras.

Chromosomes: Structures located in the nucleus of a cell that contain genes.

Chronic: Illness or condition sustained over an extended period.

Clinical breast exam: A physical examination by a trained practitioner or professional of the breast, underarm, and collarbone area, first on one side, then on the other.

Coenzyme: A molecule that interconnects with another enzyme enabling the enzyme to operate effectively in the body, and is necessary in the utilization of vitamins and minerals.

Computed tomography (CT) scanning: An imaging technique that uses a computer to organize the information from multiple X-ray views and construct a cross-sectional image of areas inside the body.

Computer-aided diagnosis (CAD): The use of special computer programs to scan mammographic images and flag areas that look suspicious.

Core needle biopsy: The use of a small cutting needle to remove a core of tissue for microscopic examination.

Corpus luteum: A small yellow body that develops within a ruptured ovarian follicle and secretes progesterone.

Corticosteroid: Steroid hormone produced by the adrenal cortex.

Cyclic breast changes: Normal tissue changes that occur in response to the changing levels of female hormones during the menstrual cycle. Cyclic breast changes can produce swelling, tenderness, and pain.

Cyst: Fluid-filled sac. Cysts are benign.

Diagnostic mammogram: The use of X rays to evaluate the breasts of a woman who has symptoms of disease such as a lump, or whose screening mammogram shows an abnormality.

Digital mammography: A technique for recording X-ray images in computer code, which allows the enhancement of subtle, but potentially significant, changes.

Diosgenin: A large steroid molecule existing in plants.

Ductal carcinoma in situ (DCIS): Cancer that is confined to the ducts of the breast tissue.

Ducts: Channels that carry body fluids. Breast ducts transport milk from the breast's lobules to the nipple.

Endocrine system: Pertains to a gland that secretes directly into the bloodstream.

Endometriosis: Growth of endometrial tissue outside the uterus.

Endometrium: The uterine lining.

Enzymes: Specific protein catalysts produced by the cells that are crucial to chemical reactions and to the structuring or synthesizing of most compounds in the body. Enzymes execute specific functions without being consumed themselves.

Excisional biopsy: The surgical removal (excision) of an area of abnormal tissue, usually along with a margin of healthy tissue, for microscopic examination. Excisional biopsies remove the entire lump from the breast.

Extract: A concentrated solid or semisolid preparation made by removing the essential and potent portion from the original substance by adding water or alcohol and evaporating the solution.

False negative (mammograms): Breast X rays that miss cancer when it is present.

False positive (mammograms): Breast X rays that indicate breast cancer is present when the disease is truly absent.

Fat necrosis: Lumps of fatty material that form in response to a bruise or blow to the breast.

Fibroadenoma: Benign breast tumor made up of both structural (fibro) and glandular (adenoma) tissues.

Fibrocystic disease: See *Generalized breast lumpiness*.

Fine-needle aspiration: The use of a slender needle to remove fluid from a cyst or clusters of cells from a solid lump.

Frozen section: A sliver of frozen biopsy tissue. A frozen section provides a quick preliminary diagnosis but is not 100 percent reliable.

Gamma-linoleic acid (GLA): An essential fatty acid, of which flaxseed oil is a good source.

Gene: Segment of a DNA molecule and the fundamental biological unit of heredity.

Generalized breast lumpiness: Breast irregularities and lumpiness, commonplace and noncancerous. Sometimes called fibrocystic disease or benign breast disease.

Genetic change: An alteration in a segment of DNA, which can disturb a gene's behavior and sometimes leads to disease.

Glycoside: A carbohydrate that metabolizes into a sugar and nonsugar.

Grain (gr): 0.065 of a gram in weight.

Gram (gm): A metric unit of weight; there are approximately 28 grams in one ounce.

Higher risk (for breast cancer): A measure of the chances of getting breast cancer when factor(s) known to be associated with the disease are present.

Hormone: A chemical substance secreted by various glands, and carried by the bloodstream, that influences cells some distance from the source of production. Hormones signal certain enzymes to perform their functions, including the regulation of specific effects on target organs and tissues.

Hormone replacement therapy: Hormone-containing medications taken to offset the symptoms and other effects of hormone loss that accompanies menopause.

Human isomolecular: Molecules from another source that are identical to human molecules such as in hormones.

Hyperplasia: Excessive growth of cells. Several types of benign breast conditions involve hyperplasia.

Hysterectomy: The surgical removal of a woman's uterus.

Immunotherapy: Techniques used to strengthen and stimulate your own immune function.

Incisional biopsy: The surgical removal of a portion of an abnormal area of tissue, by cutting into (incising) it, for microscopic examination.

Infection: Invasion of body tissues by microorganisms such as bacteria or viruses.

Infiltrating cancer: Cancer that has spread to nearby tissue, lymph nodes under the arm, or other parts of the body. Also called invasive cancer.

Inflammation: The body's protective response to injury (including infection). Inflammation is marked by heat, redness, swelling, pain, and loss of function.

International units (IU): Measurement in weight.

Intraductal papilloma: A small wartlike growth that projects into a breast duct.

Introitus: The entrance into the vaginal canal.

Invasive cancer: Cancer that has spread to nearby tissue, lymph nodes under the arm, or other parts of the body. Also called infiltrating cancer.

Laser beam scanning: A technology being studied for use in breast cancer detection. It involves shining a laser beam through the breast and recording the image produced with a special camera.

Leukocyte: A white blood cell with important functions such as destroying bacteria, fungi, and viruses and neutralizing toxins resulting from allergic reactions and cell injury.

Lobes, lobules, bulbs: Milk-producing tissues of the breast. Each of the breast's fifteen to twenty lobes branches into smaller lobules, and each lobule ends in scores of tiny bulbs. Milk originates in the bulbs and is carried by ducts to the nipple.

Localization biopsy: The use of mammography to locate tissue containing an abnormality that can be detected only on mammograms, so it can be removed for microscopic examination.

Lumpectomy: Surgery to remove only the cancerous breast lump; usually followed by radiation therapy.

Lymphatic system: The tissues and organs that produce, store, and transport cells that fight infection and disease.

Macrocalcifications: Coarse calcium deposits. They are most likely due to aging, old injuries, or inflammations and usually are associated with benign conditions.

Magnetic resonance imaging (MRI): A technique that uses a powerful magnet linked to a computer to create detailed pictures of areas inside the body.

Malignancy: State of being cancerous. Malignant tumors can invade surrounding tissues and spread to other parts of the body.

Mammary duct ectasia: A benign breast condition in which ducts beneath the nipple become dilated and sometimes inflamed; can cause pain and nipple discharge.

Mammogram: An X ray of the breast.

Mammography: The examination of breast tissue using X rays.

Mastectomy: Surgery to remove the breast (or as much of the breast as possible).

Mastitis: Infection of the breast. Mastitis is most often seen in nursing mothers.

Menometrorrhagia: Irregular and excessive menstrual bleeding.

Menopause: The time when a woman's monthly menstrual periods cease. Menopause is sometimes called the change of life.

Menorrhagia: Excessive bleeding at the time of menses, either in the number of days and/or the amount of blood lost.

Menses: Monthly flow of blood from the uterus.

Menstrual cycle: The monthly cycle of discharge, during a woman's reproductive years, of blood and tissue from the uterus.

Metrorrhagia: Uterine bleeding at a time other than the expected menses.

Microcalcifications: Tiny deposits of calcium in the breast, which can show up on a mammogram. Certain patterns of microcalcifications are sometimes a sign of breast cancer.

Microgram (mcg): 1/1,000 of a milligram in weight.

Milligram (mg): 1/1,000 of a gram in weight.

Milliliter (ml): 1/1000 of a liter.

Moon, moon time, or moon cycle: The monthly cycle of discharge, during a woman's reproductive years, of blood and tissue from the uterus.

Multiple sclerosis (MS): A disorder of the central nervous system, causing patches of sclerosis, plaques, in the brain and spinal cord, manifested by loss of normal neurological functions.

Mutation: A change in the number, arrangement, or molecular sequence of a gene.

Nanogram (ng): One-billionth of a gram in weight.

Natural killer (NK) cells: An important first line of defense; they kill infected and cancerous cells, newly arising malignant cells, and cells infected with viruses, bacteria, or protozoa.

Needle biopsy: Use of a needle to extract cells or bits of tissue for microscopic examination.

Nipple discharge: Fluid coming from the nipple.

Nonpalpable breast cancer: Cancer in breast tissue that can be seen on mammograms but cannot be felt.

One-step procedure: Biopsy and surgical treatment combined into a single operation.

Osteoporosis: A condition of mineral loss that causes a decrease in bone density and an enlargement of bone spaces, producing bone fragility.

Over the counter (OTC): A nonprescription medication.

Palpation: Use of the fingers to press body surfaces, so as to feel tissues and organs underneath. Palpating the breast for lumps is a crucial part of a physical breast examination.

Palpitations: A rapid, pounding sensation in the heart rate, which may be accompanied by an increase in anxiety.

Pathologist: A doctor who diagnoses disease by studying cells and tissues under a microscope.

Permanent section: Biopsy tissue specially prepared and mounted on slides so that a pathologist can examine it under a microscope.

Peroxides: Free radicals, by-products formed in the body when molecules of fat react with oxygen.

pH (potential of hydrogen): The degree of acidity or alkalinity of a substance or bodily aspect, such as in vaginal secretions, the intestines, or urine.

Phytochemicals: Naturally occurring chemicals produced by plants; currently, the term is being used only for those plant chemicals that may have health-related effects but are not considered essential nutrients (proteins, carbo-hydrates, fats, minerals, and vitamins). Through evolution, these plants developed new antioxidant compounds, which afforded them protection from molecules of highly reactive oxygen, enabling them to survive the oxygen pollution and slowly evolve into today's oxygen-tolerant plants. Bio-chemical defenses against bacteria, fungi, viruses, and damage to cell struc-tures, especially DNA, also became part of the plant world's arsenal. According to the American Institute for Cancer Research (newsletter 67, Spring 2000), "phytochemicals are the cancer-preventing plant chemicals abundant in a plant-based diet. For example, a cruciferous vegetable, such as broccoli, is rich in sulforaphane, a phytochemical that interferes with tumor growth; pumpkin contains carotenoids that give you protection against several cancers; capsicum, as in chili peppers, interferes with cancer development; resveratrol, in red grapes, may have a beneficial effect on blood cholesterol and help reduce the risk of skin cancer."

Phytoestrogens: "Plant" estrogens that are produced in the intestines from certain flavonoids, isoflavones (most notably genistein, biochanin A, and daidzein), and lignans. Phytoestrogens are 250 to 1,000 times weaker than human estrogen but still affect the body. Suspected of blocking estrogens by tying up estrogen receptors on cells, they thus affect hormone-related can-cers, including breast and prostate cancer. Soy foods are rich sources.

Phytogenic: Molecules of plant origin.

Phytohormones: Naturally occurring hormonelike molecules found in plants requiring no alteration in their original form or compounding action to con-vert them into hormones.

Phytosterols: Plant sterols that in modest amounts can lower cholesterol and show anticancer activity in lab and animal studies. Nuts (almonds, cashews, peanuts), seeds (sesame, sunflower), whole wheat, corn, soybeans, and many vegetable oils are good sources.

Picogram (pg): One-millionth of a microgram in weight.

Polyunsaturated: Fats or oils from vegetables, in a liquid at room temperature, are a good source of the unsaturated fatty acids. They include flaxseed, sun-flower oil, safflower oil, and primrose oil.

Positron-emission tomography (PET) scanning: A technique that uses signals emitted by radioactive tracers to construct images of the distribution of the tracers in the human body.

Postpartum: The period directly following childbirth.

Precursor: An element that precedes or converts into another.

Probiotic, originating from the Greek word for life, refers to organisms and substances contributing to healthy intestinal microbial balance and flora, the friendly intestinal bacteria.

Proliferation: Rapid reproduction of cells.

Prophylactic mastectomy: Surgery to remove a breast that is not known to contain breast cancer, for the purpose of reducing an individual's cancer risk.

Protein: Compounds essential for life, composed of hydrogen, oxygen, and nitrogen, present in the body and in foods forming complex combinations of amino acids, that are used for growth and cellular repair. Protein-rich foods include animal products, grains, legumes, and vegetables.

RAD: A unit of measure for radiation. It stands for radiation absorbed dose.

Radiation: Energy carried by waves or by streams of particles. Various forms of radiation can be used in low doses to diagnose disease and in high doses to treat disease. See *X rays.*

Radiologist: A doctor with special training in the use of X rays (and related technologies such as ultrasound) to image body tissues and to treat disease.

Risk: A measure of the likelihood of some uncertain or random event with negative consequences for human life or health.

Risk factors (for cancer): Conditions or agents that increase a person's chances of getting cancer. Risk factors do not necessarily cause cancer; rather, they are indicators, statistically associated with an increase in likelihood.

Sclerosing adenosis: A benign breast disease that involves the excessive growth of tissues in the breast's lobules.

Screening mammogram: Breast X ray used to look for signs of disease such as cancer in people who are symptom-free.

Serum: The cell-free fluid of the bloodstream. It is separated from whole blood after blood clots.

Sonogram: The image produced by ultrasound.

Specimen X ray: An X ray of tissue that has been surgically removed (surgical specimen).

Stereotactic localization biopsy: A technique that employs three-dimensional X rays to pinpoint a specific target area. It is used in conjunction with needle biopsy of nonpalpable breast abnormalities.

Steroid: An organic compound and the term applied to a large number of hormonal substances chemically related to sterols.

Surgical biopsy: The surgical removal of tissue for microscopic examination and diagnosis. Surgical biopsies can be either excisional or incisional. See *Excisional biopsy* and *Incisional biopsy.*

Tamoxifen (Nolvadex®): A hormonally related drug that interferes with the activity of estrogen. According to the National Cancer Institute (2001), "Tamoxifen has been used for more than 20 years to treat patients with advanced breast cancer. It is used as adjuvant, or additional, therapy following primary treatment for early stage breast cancer. In women at high risk of developing breast cancer, it reduces the chance of developing the disease. Tamoxifen continues to be studied for the prevention of breast cancer and in the treatment of several other types of cancer." Preliminary results from a large international trial, the International Breast Cancer Intervention Study (IBCIS), provide additional evidence that women taking Tamoxifen experienced one-third fewer breast cancers than women who took a placebo, researchers announced on March 20, 2002, at the Third European Breast Cancer Conference in Barcelona, Spain. Please note: Tamoxifen does not always prevent recurrence of breast cancer.

Thyroid: An organ essential to normal body growth in infancy and childhood; releases thyroid hormones, iodine-containing compounds that are responsible for metabolic rate; body temperature; protein regulation; fat and carbohydrate catabolism in all cells; maintenance of growth hormone release; skeletal maturation; heart rate, force, and output. They initiate many enzyme formations necessary for muscle tone and vigor.

Tinnitus: A disturbing sensation of noise—ringing, roaring, or whooshing sound; may be accompanied by a pulsation or throbbing, caused by physical conditions.

Tumor: An abnormal growth of tissue. Tumors may be either benign or cancerous.

Tumor markers: Proteins (either amounts or unique variants) made by altered genes in cancer cells that are involved in the progression of the disease.

Turgor: Refers to the normal tension in a cell, as in distension or swelling of the skin cells determined on palpation.

Two-step procedure: Biopsy and treatment done in two stages, usually a week or two apart.

Ultrasound: The use of sound waves to produce images of body tissues.

Uterus: the muscular, pear-shaped organ held in a woman's mid-pelvis, designed to carry and nourish the embryo and developing fetus once implantation has occurred.

White blood cell (WBC): A blood cell, without hemoglobin, programmed to fight foreign invaders by eliminating the foreign substance from the body.

X ray: A high-energy form of radiation. X rays form an image of body structures by traveling through the body and striking a sheet of film.

Yang: Has tonifying, energizing, and expanding qualities, considered the male aspect of balance.

Yeast: A single-cell organism that potentially causes infections vaginally, systemically, as in candidiasis, orally, dermatologically, or in the gastrointestinal tract.

Yin: Has nourishing, inward, and receptive qualities, considered the female aspect of balance.

BIBLIOGRAPHY

BOOKS

Biological Homeopathic Industries. *Homeopathic Therapy: Physicians Reference.* Albuquerque, N.M.: Menaco Publishing Co., Inc., 1990.

Boericke, William. *Homeopathic Materia Medica,* 9th edition. Arjun Nagar, New Delhi: B. Jain Publishing Co., 1974.

Coulter, Catherine. *Portraits of Homeopathic Medicines: Psychophysical Analysis of Selected Constitutional Types.* Berkeley, Calif.: North Atlantic Books, 1986.

Deal, Sheldon C. *New Life Through Nutrition.* Tucson, Ariz.: New Life Publishing, 1974.

Gaby, Alan R. *Preventing and Reversing Osteoporosis.* Rocklin, Calif.: Prima Publishing, 1995.

Gosch, Peter. *Pekana European Remedy Guide.* 1998.

Grieve, M. *A Modern Herbal.* New York: Dover Publications, Inc., 1971.

Kent, James Tyler. *Repertory of the Homeopathic Materia Medica,* 6th edition. Pahar Ganj, New Delhi: B. Jain Publishing Co., 1974.

Krochmal, Arnold, and Connie Krochmal. *A Guide to the Medicinal Plants of the United States.* New York: Quadrangle/The New York Times Book Co., 1975.

Kruzel, Thomas. *Acute Homeopathic Prescriber.* Portland, Ore.: NCNM Library, 1988.

Lee, John R. *Natural Progesterone: The Multiple Roles of a Remarkable Hormone.* Sebastopol, Calif.: BLL Publishing, 1993.

Monda, Lorena. *Golden Flower Chinese Herbs Formula Guide,* 3rd edition. Placitas, N.M.: Jin Hua Press, 1999.

Morrison, Roger. *Desktop Guide to Keynotes and Confirmatory Symptoms.* Albany, Calif.: Hahnemann Clinic Publishing, 1993.

Panos, Maesimund, and Jane Heimlich. *Homeopathic Medicine at Home.* Los Angeles: Jeremy P. Tarcher, Inc., 1980.

Rose, Jeanne. *Herbs & Things.* New York: Workman Publishing Co., 1976.

Routine Therapy, 3rd edition. Albuquerque, N.M.: Heel Biotherapeutics, 1998.

Thomas, Clayton L., ed. *Taber's Cyclopedic Medical Dictionary.* Philadelphia: F. A. Davis Co., 1993.

Tyler, M. L. *Homeopathic Drug Pictures.* London and Reading, England: The Eastern Press Ltd., 1987.

Vithoulkas, George. *Materia Medica Viva.* Mill Valley, Calif.: Health and Habitat, 1992.

Weed, Susun. *Menopausal Years.* Woodstock, N.Y.: Ash Tree Publishing, 1992.

ARTICLES

Bachmann, G. A. "Androgen Cotherapy in Menopause: Evolving Benefits and Challenges." *American Journal of Obstetrics and Gynecology* 180, no. 3, pt. 2 (March 1999): 308–311.

Ballweg, M. L. "Endometriosis: The Basics. What Is Endometriosis?" In *Overcoming Endometriosis,* M. L. Ballweg and the Endometriosis Association, eds. New York: Congdon & Weed, 1987.

Barnes, Broda. "Hypothyroidism." *Women's Health Connection,* November 1997.

Bergkvist, L., H. O. Adami, I. Persson, R. Hoover, and C. Schairer. "The Risk of Breast Cancer After Estrogen and Estrogen-Progesterone Replacement." *New England Journal of Medicine* 321 (1989): 293–297.

Braveman, Eric. "Natural Estrogen and Progesterone Research Indicates Health Benefits of Natural vs. Synthetic Hormones." *Total Health* 13, no. 5 (October 1991).

Campbell, B. C., and P. T. Ellison. "Menstrual Variation in Salivary Testosterone Among Regularly Cycling Women." *Hormone Research* 37 (1992): 132–136.

Chakmakjian, Z. "Bioavailability of Progesterone with Different Modes of Administration." *Journal of Reproductive Medicine* 32 (1987).

Chappel, S. C., and C. Howles. "Reevaluation of the Roles of Luteinizing Hormone and Follicle Stimulating Hormone in the Ovulatory Process." *Human Reproduction* 6, no. 9 (October 1991): 1206–1212.

Check, Jerome, and Harriet Adelson. "The Efficacy of Progesterone in Achieving Successful Pregnancy." *International Journal of Fertility* 32, no. 2 (1987): 139–141.

Cutson, T. M., and E. Meuleman. "Managing Menopause." *American Family Physician* 61, no. 5 (March 2000): 1391–1400, 1405–1406.

Davis, S. "Androgen Replacement in Women: A Commentary." *Journal of Clinical Endocrinology and Metabolism* 84, no. 6 (June 1999): 1886–1891.

De Cherney, A. H. "Hormone Receptors and Sexuality in the Human Female." *Journal of Women's Health* 9, supplement 1 (2000): 9–13.

Douglass, William Campbell. "A Neglected Hormone—Testosterone for Men and Women." *Second Opinion* 5, no. 3 (March/April 1995): 4.

Ellison, P. T., C. Panter-Brick, S. F. Lipson, and M. T. O'Rourke. "The Ecological Context of Human Ovarian Function." *Human Reproduction* 8 (1993): 2248–2258.

European Recombinant Human LH Study Group. "Recombinant Human Luteinizing Hormone to Support Recombinant Human Follicle Stimulating Hormone-Induced Follicular Development in LH and FSH Deficient Anovulatory Women: A Dose Finding Study." *Journal of Clinical Endocrinology and Metabolism* 83, no. 5 (May 1998): 1507–1514.

Follingstad, Alvin H. "Estriol, the Forgotten Estrogen?" *JAMA* 239, no. 1 (January 1978).

Gaby, Alan R. "Dehydroepiandrosterone: Biological Effects and Clinical Significance." *Alternative Medicine Review* 1, no. 2 (1996): 60–69.

Hargrove, Joel T., and Kevin G. Osteen. "An Alternative Method of Hormone Replacement Therapy Using the Natural Sex Steroids." *Infertility and Reproductive Medicine* 6, no. 4 (October 1995): 653–674.

Hargrove, J. T., A. C. Maxson, and L. S. Burnett. "Menopausal Hormonal Replacement Therapy with Continuous Daily Oral Micronized Estradiol and Progesterone." *Journal of Obstetrics & Gynecology* 71 (1989): 606–612.

Henderson, B. E., R. K. Ross, M. C. Pike, and J. T. Casagrande. "Endogenous Hormones as a Major Factor in Human Cancer." *Cancer Research* 42, (1982): 3232–3239.

Hileman, Beth. "Reproductive Estrogens Linked to Reproductive Abnormalities, Cancer." *Chemical and Engineering News* (January 1994): 19–23.

Hoeger, K. M., and D. A. Guzick. "The Use of Androgens in Menopause." *Clinical Obstetrics and Gynecology* 42, no. 4 (December 1999): 883–894.

Imthurn, B., A. Piazzi, and E. Loumaye. "Recombinant Human Luteinizing

Hormone to Mimic Mid-Cycle LH Surge." *Lancet* 348, no. 3 (1996): 332–333.

Johnson, Blankenschtein, and Langer. "Permeation of Steroids Through Human Skin." *Journal of Pharmaceutical Sciences* 84, no. 9 (September 1995): 1144–1146.

Kingsberg, S. A. "Postmenopausal Sexual Functioning: A Case Study." *International Journal of Fertility, Women's Medicine* 43, no. 2 (March/April 1998): 122–128.

Leary, Warren E. "Progesterone May Play Major Role in the Prevention of Nerve Disease." *The New York Times,* June 27, 1995.

Lee, J. R. "Is Natural Progesterone the Missing Link in Osteoporosis Prevention and Treatment?" *Medical Hypotheses* 35 (1991): 316–318.

———. "Osteoporosis Reversal: The Role of Progesterone." *International Clinical Nutrition Review* 10, no. 3 (July 1990).

Lees, B., T. Molleson, T. R. Arnett, and J. C. Stevenson. "Differences in Proximal Femur Density over Two Centuries." *Lancet* 341 (1993): 673–675.

Masters, W. H. "Sex and Aging—Expectations and Reality." *Hospital Practice* (August 15, 1986): 175–198.

Meston, C. M. "Aging and Sexuality." *Western Journal of Medicine* 167, no. 4 (October 1997): 285–290.

Myers, C. S., et al. "Effect of Estrogen, Androgen, and Progestin on Sexual Psychophysiology and Behavior in Postmenopausal Women." *Journal of Clinical Endocrinology and Metabolism* 70, no. 4 (1990): 1124–1131.

Naftolin, F., et al. "The Cellular Effects of Estrogens on Neuroendocrine Tissues." *Journal of Steroids and Biochemistry* 30 (1988): 195–207.

Nolan, C. R., et al. "Aluminum and Lead Absorption from Dietary Sources in Women Ingesting Calcium Citrate." *Southern Medical Journal* 87, no. 9 (September 1994): 894–898.

Prior, J. C. "Progesterone as a Bone-Trophic Hormone." *Endocrine Review* 11, no. 2 (1990): 386–398.

Prior, J. C., Y. M. Vigna, and N. Alojado. "Progesterone and the Prevention of Osteoporosis." *Canadian Journal of Obstetrics/Gynecology & Women's Health Care* 3 (1991): 178–184.

Raloff, J. "The Gender Benders." *Science News* 145 (January 1994): 24–27.

Raz, Raul, and Walter E. Stamm. "A Controlled Trial of Intravaginal Estriol in Postmenopausal Women with Recurrent Urinary Tract Infections." *New England Journal of Medicine* 329, no. 11 (September 1993): 753–756.

Redmond, G. P. "Hormones and Sexual Function." *International Journal of Fertility and Women's Medicine* 44, no. 4 (July/August 1999): 193–197.

Sarrel, P. M. "Psychosexual Effects of Menopause: Role of Androgens." *American Journal of Obstetrics and Gynecology* 180, no. 3, pt. 2 (March 1999).

———. "Effects of Hormone Replacement Therapy on Sexual Psychophysiology and Behavior in Postmenopause." *Journal of Women's Health Gender Based Medicine* 9, supplement 1 (2000): 25–32.

Schoot, D. C., J. Harlin, Z. Shoham, et al. "Recombinant Human Follicle Stimulating Hormone and Ovarian Response in Gonadotrophin Deficient Women." *Human Reproduction* 9 (1994): 1237–1242.

Sherwin, B. B., and M. M. Gelfand. "Differential Symptom Response to Parenteral Estrogen and/or Androgen Administration in the Surgical Menopause." *American Journal of Obstetrics and Gynecology* 151 (1995): 153–160.

Shoupe, D. "Androgens and Bone: Clinical Implications for Menopausal Women." *American Journal of Obstetrics and Gynecology* 80, no. 3, pt. 2 (March 1999): 329–333.

Stevenson, J. C., K. F. Ganger, et al. "Effects of Transdermal Versus Oral Hormone Replacement Therapy on Bone Density in Spine and Proximal Femur in Postmenopausal Women." *Lancet* 336 (1990): 265–326.

"Topically Applied Natural Progesterone for Relief of PMS, Pre- and Postmenopausal Conditions and Osteoporosis." *Women's Health Connection* (June 1997).

Weiss, R. "Estrogen in the Environment." *The Washington Post,* January 25, 1994.

Wilson, P.W.F., R. J. Garrison, and W. P. Castelli. "Postmenopausal Estrogen Use, Cigarette Smoking, and Cardiovascular Morbidity in Women Over 50." *New England Journal of Medicine* 313 (1985): 1038–1043.

Young, Ronald L. "Androgens in Postmenopausal Therapy?" *Menopause Management* (May 1993).

INDEX

abortion, spontaneous, 59
absent cycles, 85–88, 102, 103. *See also*
  menopause; postmenopause;
  pregnancy
abuse: self-, 36, 47, 143; verbal and
  physical, 47, 144
accident proneness, 48, 140
acidophilus, 93, 169, 171
acne: and evaluation of hormone level,
  22; and menopause, 160; and
  perimenopause, 140; and PMS, 48,
  53–54; and progesterone, 104; and
  testosterone dominance, 104–106;
  and unbalanced hormones, 36, 38,
  40; and understanding hormones,
  26, 27, 30, 33
Aconite, 90, 156, 158, 174, 186, 270,
  271, 272, 275, 292
acupuncture: and absent periods, 87;
  and breast conditions, 239; and
  DHEA, 99, 101; and
  endometriosis, 256, 258; and
  estrogen, 97; and headaches/
  migraines, 91; and heart, 191; and
  hot flashes, 188; and menopause,
  206; and ovarian cysts, 267; and
  perimenopause, 206; and PMS, 70,
  75; and postmenopause, 206; and
  pregnancy, 82; and progesterone,

82, 87, 94; and stress, 188; and
  testosterone, 108, 111; and uterine
  fibroids, 272, 276; and vaginal
  conditions, 168; and weight, 125
Adcock, Fleur, 277
addictions, 56, 152, 191, 196
Addison's disease, 33
adolescent growth, 25
adrenal exhaustion: cause of, 132; and
  compounded phytogenic hormone
  therapy, 133, 134; and DHEA
  deficiency, 99; and endometriosis,
  248, 255, 257; and estrogen, 96,
  132–36; and menstruation, 154;
  natural treatment options for,
  133–34; and pain, 132; and
  perimenopause, 139; possible
  causes of, 132; and progesterone,
  132; Rx Summary for, 134–36;
  and sex, 159; symptoms of, 33–34;
  testing for, 131; and testosterone
  deficiency, 111; and thyroid, 127,
  131; and unbalanced hormones,
  39–40; and understanding
  hormones, 33–34; and weight, 125
adrenal glands: and absent periods, 86;
  and endometriosis, 252; and
  evaluation of hormone level, 20,
  22; functions of, 33, herbal

biestrogen (*cont'd*)
    fibroids, 270, 271; and weight,
    115, 124
Bio-Botanical Research, Inc., 220, 284
Bio-Tech, 128–29
Bio-Throid, 127, 128–29, 131
biofeedback, 176
bioidentical hormones, 4
Biomed Comm, Inc., 284
biopsy, 232, 233
BIOS Biochemicals, 284–85
biotin, 82
birth control pills, 103, 228, 245–46,
    259, 261, 271
black cohosh, 64, 74, 90, 96, 107, 111,
    177, 187, 301
black current, 175, 301
black walnut leaf, 164
blackstrap molasses, 177, 197
bladder: and burning feeling, 163, 174,
    175; conditions of, 167, 174–77;
    and endometriosis, 242;
    homeopathic remedies for, 201;
    infections in, 7, 92, 162, 166, 174;
    and menopause, 160; natural
    treatments for, 174–75, 176–77;
    pain in, 201; and risks/side effects
    of synthetic estrogens, 7; and
    surgical menopause, 147
bladder wrack, 129, 220
bleeding: and evaluation of hormone
    level, 22; and unbalanced
    hormones, 38. *See also* irregular
    periods; menstruation
bloating, 36, 39, 48, 56, 63, 139, 141,
    160, 202, 243. *See also* fluid
    retention
Blood and Lymph Liquezyme, 219
blood clotting, 6, 24, 65
blood cysts, 262
Blood Liquezyme, 219
blood pressure, 7, 26, 31, 33, 34, 160,
    190, 191
blood sugar, 24, 31, 136, 139, 203
blood test, 20–21, 79, 100, 127, 153,
    189, 244
BMR formula, 129, 130
body: magnetic field of, 265

Body Ecology Diet, The, (Gates), 118
body odor, 142, 187
bones, 24, 25, 33, 38, 108, 142, 188,
    192–99. *See also* osteoporosis
Borax, 174
boric acid, 169, 170
boron, 65, 152, 194, 195, 198, 303
brain, 25. *See also* memory
breasts: abscesses in, 230, 233, 234,
    235, 238; benign conditions in,
    224, 233–37; cancer of, 6, 9, 10,
    24, 210, 211, 224, 226–27, 231,
    232, 233, 234, 235; and
    compounded phytogenic
    progesterone therapy, 232, 233,
    238; compresses and poultices for,
    226, 227, 229, 230, 231, 232,
    235–37, 239; cysts in, 225–27,
    233, 234; and estrogen, 223, 224,
    225, 233; and fat necrosis,
    231–32; fibroadenomas in,
    227–28, 233; fibrocystic, 10, 24,
    63, 224–26, 234, 235, 238; final
    note about, 239–40; herbal
    remedies for, 63, 64, 202, 228;
    homeopathic remedies for, 201,
    225, 226, 228, 229, 230, 231, 232,
    234–35, 237, 238; hormones'
    interrelationship with, 223;
    infections in, 228, 235;
    inflammation in, 228, 229–30,
    234; and intraductal papillomas,
    232, 233; and mammary duct
    ectasia, 231, 233; and mastitis,
    229–30, 234, 235, 238; and
    menopause, 160, 202, 231, 232;
    and menstruation, 85, 151, 154,
    223, 233, 235, 238; nonsurgical
    treatments for benign conditions
    in, 233–37; pain in, 126, 229, 230,
    231, 232, 234–35; and
    perimenopause, 140, 231; and
    PMS, 48, 56, 60, 63, 64; and
    progesterone, 85, 93, 223, 224,
    225, 226, 227, 228, 229, 231,
    233–34, 237, 238; and reasons for
    taking hormones, 9, 10; and risks/
    side effects of synthetic estrogens,

progesterone, 269, 270, 271, 272, 275; and reasons for taking hormones, 10; Rx Summary for, 275–76; and sleep, 180; and stress, 276; symptoms of, 268–72; and synthetic estrogens, 7; and testosterone, 270, 271, 272, 275; treatment options for, 272–75; and understanding hormones, 26; and vitamins and minerals, 276; and womb meditation, 274–75, 276

uterus: bleeding from, 147; burning feeling in, 273; contractions of, 159; hemorrhaging from, 158; and herbal remedies, 64; and meditation, 274–75, 276; and menopause, 146–47, 160; and menstruation, 155; normal, 268–72; and ovarian cysts, 268; and reasons for taking hormones, 9; structure of, 268; surgical removal of, 146–48; and synthetic estrogens, 6; tumors in, 264, 273; and understanding hormones, 25; and uterine prolapse, 147, 201, 255. *See also* endometriosis; uterine cancer; uterine fibroids

Uva Ursi, 175, 302

vagina: atrophy of, 169; burning feeling in, 163, 168; and compounded phytogenic hormone therapy, 167; conditions of, 167–73; dryness of, 141, 150, 151, 159, 162, 163, 164–65, 167–69, 171, 202, 206; and estrogen, 18; exercise for, 165–67, 205, 206; homeopathic remedies for, 202; infections in, 61, 93, 167, 169–73, 174; and menopause, 147, 160, 202, 205, 206; and menstruation, 150, 151; natural treatments for, 164–65, 168–70, 171, 172, 173; pain in, 168, 169; and perimenopause, 140, 141, 205, 206; and postmenopause, 205, 206; and progesterone, 93, 167–68, 170; and sex, 159, 162, and

testosterone, 168; and unbalanced hormones, 37, 38

valerian, 182, 187

Valerianaheels, 182, 300

verbena, 130

vervain, 91

Viburnum, 81

Victoria Apotheke Zurich, 291

violet, 187

vitamin A, 66, 74, 81, 130, 200, 258, 305

vitamin B-1, 81, 200

vitamin B-2, 81

vitamin B-3 (niacin), 130, 200, 305

vitamin B-5 (pantothenic acid), 81, 134, 200, 304

vitamin B-6 (pyridoxine), 81, 130, 134, 200, 305

vitamin B-12, 81, 129, 130, 143, 200

vitamin B-15 (pangamic acid), 134, 305

vitamin B-complex, 65, 74, 200, 205, 221, 255, 258, 305

vitamin C: for adrenal exhaustion, 134; for bones, 198; for breast conditions, 231; for endometriosis, 246, 255, 258; and estrogen, 130, 134; glossary description for, 305; for immune system, 221–22; for menopause, 205; for perimenopause, 205; for PMS, 65, 66, 74; for postmenopause, 205; for pregnancy and miscarriages, 82; and progesterone deficiency, 82; for thyroid, 130; for uterine fibroids, 271

vitamin D, 65, 74, 82, 195, 198, 258, 305

vitamin E, 59, 65, 66, 74, 82, 130, 134, 151, 164, 200, 205, 258, 305

Vitamin Express, 290

vitamin K, 82

Vitamin Research Products, 290

vitamins and minerals: for adrenal exhaustion, 134, 135; for bones, 198; for breast conditions, 239; and cancer, 221–22; and DHEA, 99, 101; for endometriosis, 246, 247, 248, 252, 255, 258; and

ABOUT THE AUTHOR

SAUNDRA MCKENNA, C.N.M., has been in private practice since 1984 in New Mexico and Hawaii. She attended Johns Hopkins University, and graduated from the College of Santa Fe and the University of California at San Francisco Nurse-Midwifery Program. She lives in La Madera, New Mexico.